AUERBACH Computer Science Series

Ned Chapin, Ph.D., General Editor

NED CHAPIN   *Flowcharts*
BARY W. POLLACK, ed.   *Compiler Techniques*
COMTRE CORPORATION, Edited by ANTHONY P. SAYERS   *Operating Systems Survey*
JOHN K. LENHER   *Flowcharting: An Introductory Text and Workbook*
J. VAN DUYN   *Documentation Manual*
ENOCH HAGA, ed.   *Computer Techniques in Biomedicine and Medicine*
RAYMON D. GARRETT   *Hospitals—A Systems Approach*

Hospitals — a systems approach

Raymon D. Garrett

First Edition

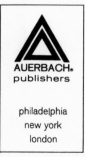

AUERBACH®
publishers

philadelphia
new york
london

AUERBACH Publishers Inc.

Philadelphia, Pa., 1973

First Printing

Printed in the United States of America

Library of Congress Cataloging in Publication Data

Garrett, Raymon D   1935-
    Hospitals--a systems approach.

    (Auerbach computer science series)
    Includes bibliographies.
    1. Electronic data processing--Hospitals--
Administration. 2. Health facilities--Planning.
I. Title. II. Series.   [DNLM: 1. Automatic
data processing. 2. Hospital administration. WX
26.5 G239h 1973]
RA971.G37 1973   362.1'1'02854   73-1686
ISBN 0-87769-156-8

Contents

v

List of Illustrations

Preface

The modern hospital has become the victim of national trends that threaten to destroy its effectiveness as a house of healing. On the one hand, a huge increase in demand for services and, on the other, an equally huge increase in paper work have overloaded the health care delivery system. Insurance companies have established stringent reimbursement rate structures in the face of exponential cost increases, and medical schools are turning out fewer physicians per capita at a time when professional personnel demands are at an all-time high.

It is the thesis of this book that good management can alleviate these problems by better allocation of resources, better use of professional time, and better availability of medical information and technology. Thus, the application of management techniques should improve the quality and quantity of medical services, and the computer is a vital adjunct to modern management techniques.

This book is intended to be read by working professionals; but if use is made of the bibliography, a senior level course could be built around this text. The book could also be used as source material for a seminar in data processing in a public health administration program.

This book grew out of a series of lectures and presentations to computer-systems and sales personnel designed to prepare them for marketing and analysis in the hospital industry. The hospital user demands a high degree of understanding of health care delivery problems. More and more users from all industries are making demands of this kind. The original intent was to provide some of the background needed to prepare sales-systems teams for marketing and installation of computers in hospitals.

As the book grew, it became clear that the material had broader appeal and value. The data-processing specialist wishing to build or further a career in hospital or medical applications would find the information of significant help in understanding the work environment.

The material is presented from the viewpoint of a systems analyst talking to other systems analysts. No attempt is made to explain computer concepts. The intended audience consists of EDP professionals. On the other hand, this is not a how-to-do-it book on hospital computer applications. The subject is the hospital, its organization, administration, and operation. We will examine hospital history, policy formation, and the kind of data involved, but always with the intent of understanding processes, not automating functions.

I do not claim originality for most of the ideas in this book. My attempt has been to compile the collective viewpoints of many professionals in the hospital field, from administrators to doctors, from consultants to computer vendors, and from small community hospitals to large university medical centers. On the other hand, the presentation is my own; and my sources must remain blameless for its faults.

I am indebted to many people, who have given their time and answered my questions patiently and unselfishly, often without knowing they were contributing to what eventually became this manuscript. Steven Saltzberg, Ida Green, J. Richardson Adams, Rubin Olsher, and many others have been directly involved in discussions concerning the topics covered in these pages. The helpful comments of Dr. Ned Chapin are evident on every page. And finally, I must mention my wife, Helen, whose honest and critical eye (and assistance with proofreading) were indispensable.

Raymon D. Garrett

Harbor City, California
May 1972

Hospitals—

a systems approach

1

Hospitals:
History and Characteristics

INTRODUCTION

The recent history of medicine exhibits striking parallels to the development of computer technology. The growth rate in both fields has been phenomenal in the past decade. Professionals in both areas have been flooded with information concerning new tools and methods at an ever faster pace. Often, before the previous materials have been digested, new ones are at hand. It has been estimated that a physician who wishes to remain up-to-date must read 30 to 40 monthly journals. EDP professionals are faced with a similar problem in the proliferation of trade and technical publications. In both computers and medicine, techniques and equipment have become essential today that did not exist ten years ago. Solutions are available to problems that were not even recognized in the 1950s.

Developments in these areas have become interdependent as well as parallel. Automation has changed medical practice to a surprising degree. Laboratory tests can be conducted, evaluated, and presented to the doctor largely without human intervention. Patient histories can be taken by computer from a teletype or CRT terminal. And the hospital business office is rare that does not utilize some degree of electronic data processing. This trend is likely to accelerate as doctors and hospital management become more familiar with the advantages of automation. Similarly, the needs of medical data processing have had a marked effect on hardware and software developments. Minicomputers were built to handle process control functions, such as are found in the clinical laboratory. Manufacturers have designed terminals and peripheral devices to the specifications of the hospital and medical service bureau. An entire computer field has grown up around the requirements of intensive, postoperative, and cardiac patient monitoring. Most large vendors have dedicated sales and systems consultants to this expanding area. These trends will also continue in the coming years.

It is not surprising, in the light of this intertwined activity, that some of the more enterprising members of both professions have seen fit to compare notes and initiate cooperative efforts for mutual benefit. A few pioneers were involved in this way from the beginning, but in recent years such efforts have become more widespread and more fruitful.

In its early stages, the computer industry was unable to offer more than the basic hardware. The machinery was welcomed in areas where manual methods could no longer handle the information-processing load. Later, computer manufacturers were induced to provide high-level languages, system monitors, and elaborate operating systems. Soon it was recognized that even these improvements could not satisfy the needs of the sophisticated user. New demands were made of the supplier of data-processing equipment and services— demands that could only be met by a "total system" approach, hardware, application programs, operating systems, and procedures.

It has taken somewhat longer than usual for the hospital/medical field to progress through these stages, perhaps because of its late start in data processing. In 1958 there were few references in the literature to biomedical or administrative hospital data processing. A few of the larger hospitals, Stamford Hospital in Connecticut, Veteran's Administration in Washington, D.C., Children's Hospital of Pittsburgh, to name a few, were experimenting with punched card systems in their business offices. By 1965 several hospital associations, notably midwestern Blue Cross organizations, were embarked on very large, complex computer systems to be shared by many hospitals. Today these are a reality. The next step is beginning to take shape. Progressive hospital data-processing people are looking for ways to integrate functions and equipment, to provide central storage and retrieval of widely used data, and to eliminate the costly duplications and opportunities for dangerous errors that exist in most manual systems. The key word is *systems* , a complete package of applications, equipment, software, training, and everything needed to satisfy the information-processing requirements.

A glance at some of the problems of the modern hospital provides insight into the strength of the demands and the force of their influence on the computer industry.

Administrative Load. The burden of paper work in the hospital has always been heavy, and the increased reporting requirements of Blue Cross, Medicare, and other insurance carriers has strained the system to the breaking point. More and more professional time is consumed by clerical duties. In addition, the extension of services offered by the large hospital has made the administrative procedures much more complex. All these factors are reflected in the flow of data within the hospital.

Patient Care. More of our citizens than ever before are demanding medical care. This is partly because the young and the aged, with their increased medical problems, make up a larger percentage of the population and partly because Medicare and the general affluence make treatment available to more people. In any event, a better-educated public is demanding more and better-quality medical care than ever in our history. To meet these demands in view of the shortages of personnel and facilities is one of the great challenges facing the modern hospital. The storage and retrieval of data are not the least part of the problem.

Expenses. Total medical expenditures in 1960 were about $20 billion. They will reach $100 billion or about 10 percent of our gross national product by 1975, an increase of 500 percent in 15 years. Some 25 percent of this figure goes to hospitals. Most of the increase in the cost of medical care is due to higher labor costs and the expensive new diagnostic and therapeutic equipment needed. An important item is the cost of processing information. About 40 percent of the total hours worked by all hospital personnel involves information handling.

The experience of other industries in cutting costs and increasing productivity by judicious application of automation suggests at least the possibility of similar benefits to be realized in hospital and medical computer applications. These expectations provide a unique opportunity for the computer industry and the data-processing professional.

Solving the information-handling problems of the hospital/medical field will require a marriage of two somewhat opposite disciplines, hospital and medical management and systems analysis. This does not imply that hospital administrators or doctors must learn computer programming, nor is it necessary that the data-processing professional acquire an MD. But a certain degree of cross-training will be vital to the kind of cooperation needed in this venture. Hospital personnel should learn something about the computer and its functions so that they may help to define their problems in terms amenable to systems treatment; and EDP specialists must become familiar with hospital operations, medical terminology, and data flow in hospital and medical management. This book is an attempt to help bridge the gap between these disciplines. It is designed primarily for the systems analyst, but several chapters could be read with benefit by hospital administrators and physicians.

In this chapter we will outline the history and growth of the modern hospital. We will discuss its purpose and charter and define its functional and organizational structure. We will attempt to remove some of the mystique of the hospital and to show that there is sense and system to this complex and confusing institution.

THE HISTORY OF THE HOSPITAL

The care of the ill and injured is an endeavor that throughout recorded history has inspired some of man's noblest efforts. Four thousand years ago in Egypt and Babylon, priests were performing surgery on battle wounds. Some of their discoveries regarding cleanliness, anesthesia, and diets were only recently reinstituted following the decline that took place during the Middle Ages. Great men, great sacrifices, and great dedication are almost commonplace in the history of medicine.

Stories of ignorance and neglect, of unnecessary suffering, of frightful death rates, of 80 percent surgical mortality, of crowded and unsanitary conditions—all these are commonplace also. The conception of the hospital as the last stop on the way to the grave is an image that has persisted for centuries, though hospitals have been improved immensely in the intervening years.

In spite of the evidence for rather advanced medical treatment by the ancients, history considers hospitals as fairly modern institutions. This view is supported by most medical historians, who classify hospital history into three phases. The first phase is the era of the almshouse, caring for all manner of sick, homeless, aged, and orphaned wanderers. The second phase involves institutions devoted to caring for the poverty-stricken who became ill or infirm. And the third, or modern, phase resulted from scientific discoveries that made hospitals the best place to care for sick people regardless of their economic condition. Though this view tends to minimize the influence and accomplishments of ancient cultures, it will be followed here for the sake of simplicity. In defense, it should be stated that we moderns did, in fact, rediscover the ancient truths of health care rather than borrow them from our predecessors without credit. Only very recent archaeological finds have shown the truly vast debt that medical science owes to ancient peoples.

The history of medicine and scientific discovery is one important facet of the history of the hospital. Social and political history is another facet, for hospitals reflect social attitudes and political realities concerning the status of the poor and sick in society. Religious history offers still another aspect of the history of the hospital, since the monastic and nursing orders played such a large part in the founding and operation of hospitals and indeed are active still. In order to describe the history of the hospital in any comprehensive way, we would have to review the entire progress of civilization. Some observers hold that a meaningful measure of the degree of civilization attained by a culture is the manner in which its members care for their sick people.

For our purposes, this view is too large. We wish to understand the operation of the modern hospital, and to do so we need to know something about the steps that led to its present structure. Thus, we will examine a few of the developments of the early phases, but most of our attention will be focused on the discoveries and developments having the greatest impact on the modern hospital: those of the late nineteenth century and of the last 50 years.

It is often stated that the status of the early hospital in Western culture was that of a charitable institution. A more accurate statement might be that the charitable institutions of pre-1900 communities served some of the functions of the modern hospital by default, since there were no hospitals, by modern standards, prior to the twentieth century. This statement is subject to the same reservations noted above concerning Babylon and Egypt, but it could be supported if we include in our definition of *hospital* the sophisticated tools available to modern physicians, products of radiology, bacteriology, microscopy, and so forth. In any event, the poorhouses, almshouses, and leper colonies were truly charitable institutions that were built by various religious and municipal agencies to care for the wandering pilgrims, the indigent infirm, and the dangerously contagious. One suspects on reading the descriptions of these early institutions that the aims of their supporters were more closely related to the quarantine of undesirables than to charitable good works. One should not, however, belittle the dedication and loving spirit that pervaded those who served and toiled within their walls to bring some measure of relief to the suffering.

The most striking characteristic of medical care in those early times was the sharp distinction between the care available to the poor and the well-to-do. The charity institution typically had no full-time physicians. Doctors donated their time as they chose, and patients were treated by whichever doctor happened to be present on the wards. The quality of treatment was severely limited by the resources of the institution. Economically solvent patients, on the other hand, were treated in the home, the conditions being determined, in a relative sense, by their wealth. We must stress *relative* because in those days before Lister and Pasteur, the best medical care money could buy was none too good. Surgery was a risky business, to be attempted only as a last resort. Patients often were maimed or killed by the infection and shock resulting from successful surgery. Nothing need be said of the unsuccessful.

The early hospital tended to become very crowded. Patients were accepted only when their complaints had reached crisis proportions. The indifferent medical care available—and the overcrowded conditions and all that they implied concerning cross infection and overworked staff—did not allow for a good prognosis for the average hospital patient. Mortality rates of 25 percent of all admissions were not uncommon. For maternity cases, the figure was closer to 50 percent; and few mothers and newborn babies left the hospital without a disease or defect acquired while in the hospital's care.

These facts reflect several conditions in society beyond the simple lack of medical knowledge and hospital facilities. It must be remembered that these were plague years, years of famine in many parts of the world, years of wars and revolutions—in other words, a time in which life itself was risky. Hospitals were no worse than society in general, and in many cases they were better. Conditions in the hospital ward were often more sanitary and less crowded than in the patients' homes. The fact is that hospitals did not have the resources or the power to stem this tide of human misery. Several changes in societal attitudes and governmental responsibilities, as well as advances in medicine, were needed to alter these conditions.

Every schoolboy is familiar with the name of Louis Pasteur, whose work in preventive medicine won him international fame. His major contribution was in the discovery that each disease has its own microorganism. This idea was not new, but Pasteur was one of the first to provide demonstrable proof using the microscope. He was also the first to use this idea for man's benefit. By allowing microbe disease cultures to degenerate and become weaker, he could develop a strain that would induce immunity to the parent disease.

From the work of Pasteur, Donne, and others, Joseph Lister, a surgeon in Glasgow, Scotland, concluded that the terrible infections occuring in post-surgical patients were due to microbes. At that time, hospital gangrene was killing some 45 percent of amputation patients. Lister experimented with several chemicals, finally settling on carbolic acid as a disinfecting agent for the air, surgical instruments, dressings, and even his hands. The results were phenomenal. Conscientious application of Lister's methods virtually eliminated infection as a major cause of death in surgery, and surgical mortality rates dropped from 80 percent to 6 percent.

Other discoveries followed in rapid succession: surgical techniques, antibiotics, X-ray diagnostics, and many others. Medicine capitalized on the resurgence of science during the latter part of the nineteenth, and the early twentieth, centuries. Now that the causes of disease were known, medical research could focus on methods for treating them effectively. In this burst of discovery, the modern hospital was born. The quality of care available to the hospital patient was greatly improved. Cleanliness alone made a great difference in the results of hospitalization.

For some time, the charity hospital had been the locus of good medical education. Only in the hospital could the student find sufficient variety in case material for an adequate grounding in medical and surgical techniques. In addition, only in a large hospital could a researcher find an adequate patient base for his studies. As the effects of Pasteur's and Lister's work took shape, the facilities and equipment in the hospital began to outstrip anything the physician could provide outside.

All these factors combined to make hospitalization more desirable for all critically ill patients, even the well-to-do. Physicians began bringing their private, paying patients, and those patients began to lose the fear of being hospitalized. The reputation of the hospital had improved in a span of about 25 years to that of a respected medical institution providing the best health care society had to offer.

Social attitudes were changing at the same time. As long as poverty and sickness were adjudged fit punishment for the sinful, little help could be expected in caring for those afflicted with disease. Indeed, we might be trespassing on divine territory by attempting to ameliorate merited suffering. If, however, human suffering is seen to be less a matter of morals than of accident and if we see that the good are stricken down with the bad, then kindness and care will pour more freely. Popular attitudes in these matters have vacillated throughout history and in different parts of the world. As these attitudes vary, so do their manifestations in terms of personal and governmental involvement, both on a local and a national or international level. The public demand for better medical care and for governmental responsibility in hospital matters was increasing at about the time of the great medical discoveries. Again, these were only part of the social milieu, one of the many areas of public concern in an age of political upheaval and rising public expectations; but the result was better funding, higher standards, and more control over the founding and operation of hospitals.

Two features separate the development and growth of hospitals in the United States from those of their European counterparts. The first has to do with initial funding and building. Seventy percent of the funds used in building American hospitals before the Depression of 1932 came from private donors. Their names read like an early social register: Hopkins, Vanderbilt, Whitney, Rockefeller. A great deal of money was collected from the general population as well. Most European hospitals were built with government funds, as are most American hospitals today, with 70 percent of the money now coming from taxation.

The other feature characteristic of American hospitals is the early move toward paying patients. As early as 1750, hospitals in the English colonies were accepting fees for services. The effect was to remove the social stigma of hospitalization and to encourage the use of the hospital by the affluent middle class. In this way, the progress of the hospital was quickened in this country. Nevertheless, a good many admissions were of poor people, and this situation still remains. Today the various levels of government in the United States pay about half of all hospital costs. In European countries the figure is closer to 95 percent.

Many factors have added impetus to the growth and expansion of modern hospitals. Among these were health insurance plans, the growth of professional societies such as the American College of Surgeons and the American Hospital Association, and the federal Hill-Burton bill for the construction of hospitals. These provided badly needed funds and professional standards of excellence at a time when hospitals were feeling the pinch of donor funding reductions. We shall see in later chapters how these factors continue to influence hospital operations.

The role of the community hospital has increased in stature. The emphasis has changed from crisis intervention and care for the bedridden to preventive medicine, social services, and outpatient care. More and more, the hospital is becoming a community institution. Its role in society and its sense of its own mission are changing. Health care was looked upon for centuries as a boon, a charitable good work, given to the needy as humanitarian benevolence. Today we find a recognition of health as a natural right of every human being. In 1946 the World Health Organization proclaimed this right and the responsibility of signatory governments to provide it. We are beginning to see local governments, private and community hospitals, and the federal government work toward ways to implement good health for the entire population.

TYPES OF HOSPITALS

Hospitals are classified according to funding or controlling agency, services offered, and size or number of beds. These categories are useful in determining the administrative complexity, the financial difficulties, and the expected patient load.

Sponsorship or control of hospitals is particularly important in determining the administrative setting. We shall see in the next chapter that generalizations concerning procedures and management methods can be made only within a sponsorship category. These categories are federal, voluntary, church, state or local government, and proprietary. Federal hospitals are all United States Army, Air Force, and Navy hospitals; Veterans Administration hospitals; and the institutions operated by the Public Health Service, federal prisons, and the Bureau of Indian Affairs. There are about 420 of these hospitals with a total of 170,000 beds.

Voluntary hospitals consist of all privately owned, nonprofit community hospitals, by far the largest group in the United States. They number some 3,900 hospitals with about 560,000 beds.

Church hospitals are owned and operated by the various Catholic nursing orders, such as Sisters of Charity and Sisters of Mercy; the Lutheran Hospital Association, the Baptist Hospital Association, and other Protestant groups; and a small number of Jewish and LDS hospitals in certain regions. There are about 1,000 hospitals in this group with some 150,000 beds.

State, county, city, and district hospitals are paid for by taxes and usually operate on a charity basis. They currently number about 1,700 hospitals with 200,000 beds and are the fastest growing segment of the hospital field.

Proprietary hospitals are those institutions operated by private groups or corporations for a profit. There are less than 1,000 of these hospitals with only about 50,000 beds. Table 1.1 summarizes some of the pertinent facts concerning hospital ownership.

The American Hospital Association divides hospitals according to the kind of service or treatment offered. These classes are short-term general; long-term or convalescent; and psychiatric, tuberculosis, or other specialty. It is possible to break down these categories still further. Some short-term general hospitals restrict admissions to children and to maternity or orthopedic cases. Others admit only patients with eye, ear, nose, and throat complaints. In addition, there are a few rehabilitation centers and geriatric hospitals that do not fit well into

Table 1.1
Hospital ownership in the United States

Control	Number	Beds (X1,000)	Admissions (X1,000)	Expenses (X1 mil)	Assets (X1 mil)	Personnel (X1,000)
Federal	420	170	1,500	$1,600	$1,900	130
Voluntary	3,900	560	15,000	8,800	13,300	930
Church	1,000	150	5,000	3,000	4,400	370
State and local gov't.	1,700	200	6,000	3,600	4,800	400
Proprietary	750	50	1,800	800	600	80
Total	7,770	1,130	29,300	$17,800	$25,000	1,910

Table 1.2
Hospital service types

Class	Number	Beds (X1,000)	Admissions (X1,000)
Short-term general	6,000	900,000	29,100,000
Convalescent	85	50,000	260,000
Special	820	680,000	760,000

any of the usual categories. Table 1.2 summarizes the number and sizes of the hospitals in these categories.

The number of beds is one of the many convenient ways of describing hospital size. Another might be square feet of floor space or annual rate of admissions or number of nursing personnel. Hospital planners traditionally have used beds-per-1,000 population as a way of ascertaining community health needs. There is a growing realization that the services performed by a hospital in community mental health programs, emergency treatment, outpatient clinical activity, and preventive medicine—all requiring no beds at all—are equally important to the total community health delivery system. Still, as a measure of certain hospital functions and needs, bed size remains the only reliable gauge. The following table shows regional distribution of hospitals by the number of beds in the United States. The regions used are United States government census divisions:

Division 1. New England (Conn., Me., Mass., N.H., R.I., Vt.)

Division 2. Middle Atlantic (N.J., N.Y., Pa.)

Division 3. South Atlantic (Del., D.C., Fla., Ga., Md., N.C., S.C., W.Va., Va.)

Division 4. East North Central (Ill., Ind., Mich., O., Wis.)

Division 5. East South Central (Ala., Ky., Miss., Tenn.)

Division 6. West North Central (Ia., Kan., Minn., Mo., Neb., N.D., S.D.)

Division 7. West South Central (Ark., La., Okla., Tex.)

Division 8. Mountain (Ariz., Colo., Id., Mont., Nev., N.M., Ut., Wyo.)

Division 9. Pacific (Alas., Cal., Haw., Wash., Ore.)

Table 1.3
Regional distribution of hospitals by number of
beds in the United States

Division	Beds		
	0-99	100-299	300 and Over
New England	220	150	100
Middle Atlantic	300	400	320
South Atlantic	600	320	220
East North Central	570	500	300
East South Central	390	160	80
West North Central	690	230	130
West South Central	800	230	110
Mountain	350	100	50
Pacific	600	280	130
Total	4520	2370	1440

The numbers in the tables have been gathered from various publications of the American Hospital Association, the United States Public Health Service, *Modern Hospital Magazine,* and other sources. All figures were compared, and a great deal of variation was found. This is because all these agencies must depend on the responses of the hospitals themselves, and responses are not always forthcoming within the publication deadline. The figures shown are approximate and are intended to show trends and basic characteristics. It is impossible to obtain a complete and accurate census of American hospitals on a voluntary reporting basis.

Some interesting trends are observable from a study of the above tables and similar figures from past years. Hospitals are growing in size, but not very much in total numbers. It has been estimated that over 40 percent of all hospital beds will be in hospitals of over 500 beds by 1980. Small hospitals are being enlarged, absorbed in larger units, or taken out of operation.

At the same time, it is obvious that the larger hospitals will be able to provide more complete facilities, since high utilization is required to justify expensive equipment. Multiphasic screening units, specialized diagnostic and treatment apparatus, and high-level medical automation are very costly.

These larger medical centers, combining the latest equipment with the highest utilization, can exist only in the large metropolitan areas. A study of geographical distribution demonstrates the accuracy of this prediction. Over 60 percent of the larger hospitals are found along the Eastern seaboard.

One additional fact of interest is that proprietary hospitals, those operated for profit, are growing in size and shrinking in number, following the general trend. This is of importance to the computer specialist, since one of the characteristics of the management of proprietary hospitals is a stronger commitment to cost consciousness, thus increasing the interest of such institutions in computer applications.

DEFINITIONS AND DESCRIPTIONS
OF THE HOSPITAL

General Viewpoint

There are many ways to define or describe the nature of the modern hospital. It may be looked upon as part of the community health care delivery system. It may be viewed as an organizational entity of particular complexity. A functional description may be given or a systems viewpoint adopted. All of these are valid and useful ways of discussing a very complicated subject. The hospital has facets reflecting all these views, and a closer look from each of these vantage points can be instructive.

Health and the Community

The administration of community resources has received a great deal of attention in recent years, particularly as an informed and vocal public insists upon obtaining certain services from community government. These services include utilities, fire and police protection, library services, parks and recreation, and health services. Health as a personal ideal has been valued by most people everywhere, but in Western countries in the last 50 years there has been a growing demand for unified action in areas where individuals cannot or might not be effective. Communicable diseases, preventive medicine, chronic and vocational illnesses, and mental health are all areas in which public agencies have operated with great success. One need only mention the diphtheria and smallpox epidemics of a century ago and compare them to the recent conquests of tuberculosis and polio to demonstrate this success.

Along with the scientific advances and great strides in medical progress, there has been a realization of the social and economic relationships influencing public health. Availability of community resources such as sewage control and clean water, medical and hospital services, and protection from communicable diseases had been in the past too often a function of the economic condition of a neighborhood, with results that were dangerous to everyone in the community. It is evident that we can be only as safe and as healthy as our neighbors.

The response of community government in most areas has been to attempt to develop cooperative planning and action councils to coordinate the many commercial enterprises, voluntary associations, and governmental agencies at all levels that are involved in community health. To list these organizations in a large city and to outline their interrelationships and independent activities is to begin to understand the size and complexity of the coordinating task. Insurance companies, drug dispensaries, and most professional medical and dental services are run by private enterprise, with minimal governmental involvement. Most hospitals, home nursing services, medical research, foundations, and community health agencies are voluntary nonprofit corporations. And environmental sanitation, health education, vital statistics, mental health, and communicable disease control are a few of the jobs performed by public health agencies of city, county, state, or federal governments.

The place of the hospital as part of this community health services complex is of interest to us in our study of hospital operations. This question leads naturally to a discussion of the functions of a hospital. Without preempting the next section, we can divide these functions into three areas as they relate to care of the ill and the injured in society: inpatient care, outpatient care, and home nursing.

The first of these is the traditional province of the acute short-term general hospital; but public demand has encouraged a broader role, especially for large city hospitals. Though physicians continue to serve medical needs on an individual basis, the modern general hospital has become the central source of application of medical science for many communities. Thus, the hospital must play a central role in community planning of health care. In a large community, the coordination of activities and services of many hospitals with varied plans and goals becomes a necessity if the needs of the area are to be met without waste or inadequacy. More than any other part of the health care delivery system, the modern hospital represents medical care to the people of the community.

Hospital Functions

Louis Pasteur is quoted as saying that the aim of medical practice is "to cure sometimes, to alleviate often, to comfort always." The modern hospital has adopted that sentiment as its creed. To provide the maximum health care possible consistent with its resources is the goal of the hospital, whether it is governed by a private, a voluntary, or a governmental body. Health care, as it is provided by hospitals, can be viewed as the result of six basic activities: diagnosis, therapy, rehabilitation, prevention, education, and research. The modern hospital is active to some degree in all these areas as it fulfills its role in community health.

As a part of the community health care delivery system, the hospital is deeply involved in the prevention of disease and the detection and control of epidemics. A great deal of effort is expended to control contagion from outside sources and cross infection of patients in the hospital. It is also important to insure against infection spreading from the hospital into the community. Inoculation programs, communicable disease reporting, warnings of specific public health dangers, maintenance of quarantine areas where required—all are portions of the hospital's activity in preventive medicine.

Sometimes all preventive measures fail, and a person becomes ill. The sick person cannot be treated effectively until the nature and cause of his illness are known and the extent of the damage is evaluated. Such diagnostic data are collected by many means, some mechanical, some biochemical, some radiological, and some manual. The exact procedures vary with the judgment of the physician as he analyzes his observations, the history of the complaint, and the evidence provided by the tests he has ordered. For much of the diagnostic procedure, the doctor needs no equipment other than his hands, eyes, and ears. Other more specialized procedures require complex and expensive apparatus. Few doctors can afford to maintain clinical laboratory equipment and X-ray machines for the small number of patients they treat. The work load of one or even several physicians would not justify such an expense, nor would this be an effective use of community resources. Idle equipment almost always implies inadequate care for someone in the community.

Enter the community hospital. With hundreds of physicians and the thousands of patients they treat all coming to the same place for complicated diagnostic procedures, the utilization of equipment remains high and the cost is relatively low. Most general community hospitals maintain elaborate diagnostic departments. In performing these services, the hospital is providing one of its most valuable functions in community health.

Therapy is defined as a treatment designed to eliminate a disease or disorder of the body. Technically, therapy cannot begin until a diagnosis is known, but in practice some kind of therapy begins almost as soon as the patient enters the hospital. This is especially true in emergency situations. Therapy includes activities performed by doctors, nurses, and medical technologists. Much of this activity is carried out the same way that it was 50 or 100 years ago. On the other hand, a significant portion of activity reflects advancements and discoveries made in the last ten years. The changes in therapeutic methods, as well as the costs in time, manpower, and equipment these changes require, force a continual updating of hospital procedures and a corresponding investment of resources.

After an illness or injury has run its course, its victim must be returned to an active, useful life. Often, the disease will have made the continuance of a previous job or career impossible. Sometimes, as in coronary cases, extended bed rest is required. A variety of rehabilitative programs must be provided by the community, including long term nursing, physical therapy, occupational therapy, and the like. The large community hospital is one of the most frequent sources of these services. In some cases, it is the only source.

Because of its position as the locus of community health care, the hospital serves as a test bed and data base for a large percentage of the medical research carried out in this and other countries. Virtually all research projects, at some stage, reflect data collected from hospital patients or utilize hospital facilities to verify results. In fact, no research effort is considered complete unless clinical evidence for its findings can be cited.

In addition to the direct patient care activities described above, the community hospital is involved in three general types of educational tasks. The first of these is the obvious one of training health care professionals, the physicians, nurses, and medical technologists that staff our hospitals and clinics. Many hospitals are connected with medical schools, and hundreds maintain accredited nursing schools. The second area involves training public health and health administration personnel as part of an organized intern program or in seminars given to upgrade public health officials. Finally, a considerable amount of public instruction in health and sanitation is carried out using hospital personnel and facilities.

It is hoped that the result of all these activities will be a healthier populace. At the very least, the less fortunate can be cared for. Hospital resources are allocated with the intention of maximizing the quality and quantity of health care delivered. These resources come from society, and the public has come to expect efficiency and excellence in their use.

The hospital field is filled with men and women of dedication and devotion to these ideals. In the face of long hours and less than handsome pay, they continue to serve an increasing patient load with increasingly scarce resources. Without these selfless people, the hospital could not perform its functions.

Organization

We will devote an entire chapter to this subject later, but a brief description here is helpful. The general short-term voluntary community hospital will be used throughout this book as the model for administrative structure. There are many good reasons for this. Such hospitals are, by far, the most numerous. Their structure has been studied more than any other. Moreover, the greatest activity in data processing in this decade can be expected to take place in the community hospital.

The organization chart shown in figure 1.1 is typical of the structure of

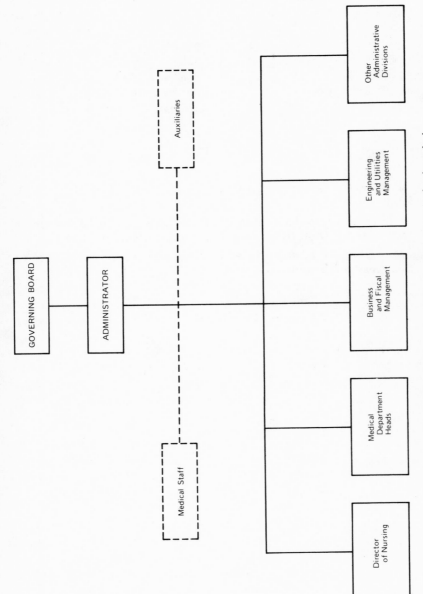

Figure 1.1   Organization chart of a typical community hospital

voluntary hospitals. The governing board is the ultimate financial and legal authority, playing much the same role as a board of directors in industry. The board hires an administrator who functions as the chief executive officer of the hospital. He, in turn, enlists the support of several paid and voluntary assistants to manage specialized departments and functions in the hospital. The administrator is also the titular head of the medical staff and auxiliary organizations working in the hospital. We shall see that this simplified picture is not an accurate or complete description of the power structure and decision-making activity in the hospital, but for our present purposes it will suffice.

REFERENCES

Crichton, Michael. *Five Patients—The Hospital Explained.* New York: Alfred A. Knopf, 1970.

Jackson, Laura G. *Hospital and Community—Studies in External Relationships of the Administrator.* New York: The Macmillan Company, 1964.

Risley, Mary. *House of Healing—The Story of the Hospital.* Garden City, N.Y.: Doubleday & Company, 1961.

2

The Hospital System

INTRODUCTION

From a systems viewpoint, the organization chart or lines-of-authority approach to the hospital is not a fruitful one. Data flow does not always follow departmental lines. The unique position of the staff physician in determining patient care activities—and thus the kind, amount, and disposition of patient data—gives him a preferred status in the hospital data management system that does not appear in the organization chart.

The systems approach to hospital operation tends to ignore the functional and departmental divisions of the hospital in favor of an information flow division. Hospital activities are treated in terms of the kind of data generated, the amount of data, the processing required, the uses made of the data, and so forth. In other words, the hospital is considered to be a set of nodes in a data flow diagram. Each node requires input of information, performs some processing, perhaps generates new data, and produces output that moves on to some other node. The nodes are chosen in a way that will clarify the procedures involved and still preserve some relationship to the usual functional view of hospital operations. This is important because as we develop an information model of the hospital, we wish to be able to utilize what we learn in improving data flow and other operations in the real hospital. We must be able to recommend changes in some hospital activities and to couch these changes in terms understandable to the hospital world. Thus the subsystems chosen will not be quite as arbitrary as they may appear.

A system may be defined as a set of things so related as to form a unit with recognizable inputs and outputs. Consonant with its purposes, the resources of the system are brought to bear on the input to produce the output. The basic assumption of systems analysis is that an understanding of the operation of a system can be derived from a study of the input/output and of the internal processing done by the system. In this view, the hospital itself is a system of which the input is sick people, the output is well people, and the internal processing includes the range of diagnostic, therapeutic, and rehabilitative procedures discussed above.

It would be possible to amplify our approach to the hospital to include this "people" input, as well as other types, supplies, visitors, and so forth. However, since our overall objective is related to data processing, we will restrict ourselves to information flow except where it becomes necessary to discuss the movement of people, supplies, and equipment to clarify the reasons for, and the nature of, the flow. It is hoped that readers unfamiliar with the systems approach will be compensated for their efforts in reading the following material by its success in clarifying the interrelationships between hospital functional areas. The aim will be to develop an overall view of hospital activities that will be made precise by the necessary detail of a systems analysis. The result should be a unifying principle, a guide to hospital operations that will be at the same time a description of present procedures, a suggestion for automating some of them, and a road map for implementing the automation.

This chapter will be devoted to a discussion of the systems approach to hospital operations. The six systems chosen reflect the kind of internal processing involved more than the function performed for the hospital. Thus, we find maintenance and clerical activities classified together, since both are basically service activities, performing little or no internal processing of information. Similarly, clinical services are classified with nursing services, not because both are patient-oriented, but because the data generated by them are almost identical. Of these six systems, five are more or less independent of each other, the sixth supplying the link that connects them and integrates the hospital into a functional unit. We will treat the first five in some detail and then attempt to unify them into an overall picture with the sixth.

No single authority is followed in this chapter, though a number of studies have been conducted using a similar approach. Two of these, Roy Hudenberg's *Planning the Community Hospital* and a Public Health Service Research Project reported in *Planning for Hospitals—A Systems Approach*, are valuable complementary reading.

The six systems are shown in figure 2.1, in which the communications system is shown integrating all hospital functions. We shall examine each system briefly and consider a few of the common applications of computers to solving relevant problems.

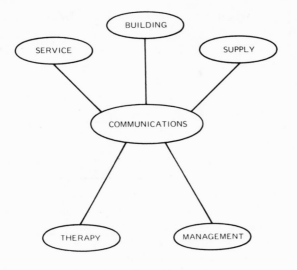

Figure 2.1   The hospital system

THE SERVICE SYSTEM

The service areas are those dedicated to performing the routine jobs necessary to the operation of the hospital, but whose activities are not crucial to the information processing tasks. Examples are the common clerical services, building maintenance, security, the library, reception, the chaplaincy, social service, and the various auxiliaries.

From an information systems viewpoint, the service system makes minimal contributions. About the only input to the system are the instructions and orders concerning services to be performed. The purpose of a service group is to perform assigned tasks, usually tasks that do not generate of themselves any significant data beyond the fact that the tasks were performed. Internal information processing consists of interpreting orders, hardly an important information system function. Output is similarly restricted, consisting of such service-oriented data as hours worked, tasks completed, and so forth. Figure 2.2 illustrates data flow in the service system.

It is a fairly easy matter to automate the usual time card and clock procedures. If a plastic card or badge is issued to each employee, positive identification is assured. A recording badge reader located at the various stations in the hospital would allow the simultaneous entry of time, work station, and badge number at the beginning and end of each work period. Tapes from these devices could be collected and processed daily for complete control of personnel

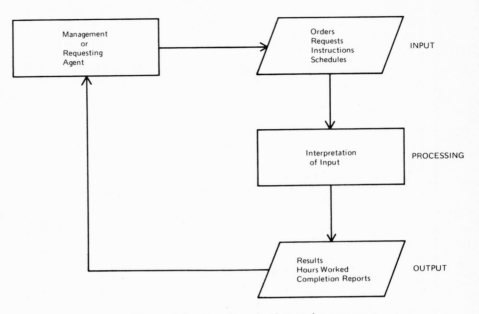

Figure 2.2   Data flow in the service system

hours worked. A similar device hooked to a computer on-line in this case, could detect the presence of doctors in the hospital.

One of the many difficult scheduling jobs in a hospital involves the preventive maintenance required by the large number of mechanical and electronic devices. Regular inspection, cleaning, lubrication, and so forth, are musts for much of this apparatus. Personnel training and turnover problems complicate the job, and the great variety of machines dictate that printed instructions must accompany each task.

A simple way to accomplish the goals of this application is to store a list of maintenance instructions on tape for each piece of equipment in the hospital, along with a frequency-of-maintenance statement. The computer can scan this tape on a monthly basis, analyze frequency of repairs and date of last maintenance to arrive at a list of equipment to be inspected during the coming month, and print out a work schedule and instructions for the plant supervisor.

THE BUILDING SYSTEM

The building system refers to the environmental control, power and utilities, and building engineering functions of the hospital, all areas pertaining to the physical plant not already included in the service system. Most inputs for this system are from analog sensor and recording instruments, humidity, temperature, pressure, and so forth. Processing is a matter of comparing readings with desired or optimum operational parameters; and output consists of a set of instructions for changes in switch, valve, or potentiometer settings to bring the various measured values into accord with the charts. These instructions are given to one of the service areas for immediate attention. A typical flow chart for building system data is given in figure 2.3.

The purpose of a building control automation system is to cut labor costs, to improve operating efficiency of primary building systems, and to minimize repairs to expensive equipment. All these purposes are served by a central control that allows one man to monitor the entire building, adjusting operating parameters, starting and stopping equipment remotely, and dispatching maintenance personnel to problem areas before complications set in.

These functions have existed in building control systems for years. The important new aspect is the ability to automate much of the monitoring and decision making by use of a digital computer. Thus, start-stop schedules, adjustments, temperature and pressure alarms, and so forth, may be programmed by the operator. Only alarm conditions or changes in operating plans would necessitate human intervention. Of course, it would be possible to override computer decisions at any time. It is also noteworthy that the demands on a computer by such a system, even for a large building, would not utilize the entire capacity of the machine. Thus, it would be feasible to share this computer with some other activities.

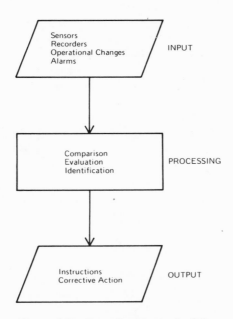

Figure 2.3   Data flow in the building
              system

THE SUPPLY SYSTEM

Two distinct areas are included in the supply system: the pharmacy and all other supply departments. In "other" are included the central medical supply, sterile supply, food, and all delivery functions. The pharmacy is set apart because of its special data-handling problems. The pharmacy acts as its own purchasing department in most hospitals, going through the business office's accounts payable section, but not dealing with the ordering, receiving, and vendor control. Drugs prescribed by the medical staff are often manufactured by the large hospital pharmacy. This is especially true of parenteral solutions. Since some 7,000 drugs are available to the doctor, a major part of the pharmacist's efforts is involved with catalogs of drugs, contraindications, dosages, and so forth, for distribution to the medical staff.

Input, to the pharmacy, consists of drug orders or prescriptions and patient record summaries. The latter allow the pharmacist to audit the kind and amount of drugs being given to the patient. Two facts make an audit vital to the patient's health. First, drugs have effects in combination with other drugs or treatments not always known to the average doctor. Secondly, a patient may be seeing several doctors who may prescribe the same drug independently, the total of which would be an overdose. It is the pharmacist's responsibility to notice this fact and to inform the physicians in question. Thus, internal processing involves screening both drug and patient data and searching for prescription or transcription errors, patient identification errors, possible contraindications, overdoses, and so forth. Output is simply charge data for the accounting department along with the occasional physician alarm.

It must be noted that drug inventories, reorders, and so forth are also done by this supply area. Deliveries are handled in some hospitals by special personnel; in others, delivery is taken care of by the normal hospital service.

All supply areas are concerned with the basic order quantities, reorder levels, and other parameters involved with modern inventory management and stock replenishment. They are also concerned with the delivery of bulk and nonbulk supply items as requested and with the proper accounting for those items that are chargeable to patients or departments. In this sense, the supply system is not different in any significant way from its industrial counterpart.

Inventory management is the science of maintaining and procuring goods while providing service to the users who place demands against those goods. *Service* means having the right item available at the right time and place. Doing this in a rapidly changing environment means the continuous calculation of the fundamental quantities of inventory control, the safety stock, the reorder point, and the economic order quantity. These values depend on carrying charges, discounts, unit costs, item demand forecasts, and so forth.

A good inventory control system will accept data from the order-processing system, update inventory quantities on hand, and record this activity for use by the forecasting programs. Each month this program will establish for each item of inventory a forecast of expected usage for the next and future months based on past activity and growth trend data, along with any seasonal or special information provided by management. A separate program then calculates updated values for SS, ROP, and EOQ for each item. These quantities become part of the report issued to management to assist in setting policies for purchasing and stores.

The screening of prescriptions for sensitivities or allergies, contraindications, and overdoses is a task of almost impossible magnitude in a hospital pharmacy without some kind of automation aids. Thousands of orders are processed each day by the medium-sized hospital. There is simply no time to examine manually the medical record of each patient receiving a drug.

A computer system can perform this task with relative ease once a few ground rules are set and a data base established. The data required are of two kinds: (1) data on each drug in the formulary with usual or maximum doses, contraindications, and possible drug interactions and (2) patient-oriented drug data that include a record of what is being taken, likely allergic reactions, diagnosis, and so forth.

Along with this data must go the procedural assurances that no drug will

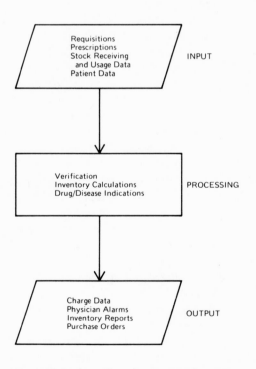

Figure 2.4 Data flow in the supply system

be given without the following of an order procedure that at some stage interacts with the computer. It is then a simple matter to scan each order against the patient, check for any situation that might contraindicate the present prescription, and notify the pharmacist and/or physician of these conditions. As in all cases involving patient-doctor relations, the doctor must make the final decision. The purpose of the system is not to control prescriptions, but to provide vital information.

THE MANAGEMENT SYSTEM

The administration of a hospital or any large organization can be divided into two separate, but dependent, functions: (1) policy and decision making and (2) financial management. Both of these areas must depend on each other for information, and both have a common interface with the rest of the hospital, so that it makes sense to speak of these two areas as a single management system.

The fiscal services include all the basic accounting functions, receivables, payables, purchasing, billing, credit and collections, payroll, and the like. These, together with auditing, form the financial management of the hospital. They are dependent on the administrative area for policy and direction. On the other hand, much of the data upon which decisions are based comes from the accounting department. The data flow through this part of the system can be simplified as indicated in figure 2.5.

Data flow in the policy formation area is not so simple. Input consists of reports, observations, conversations, and so forth, concerning the operation of the hospital; and output consists of a set of policy decisions and more or less detailed instructions on how to implement the decisions. So far so good. But the internal processing that manipulates the input and produces the output is complex enough to deserve several books. We have room for only a single short chapter, but even there the complexity will become apparent. For our purposes here, it is sufficient to say that the character of the input has some relation to the character of the output, but not in the simple way that it does in other parts of the hospital.

Opportunities for automation of management-oriented functions have been realized more than for any other hospital activity. The similarities to management activities in other industries have made this a predictable development. The common elements of accounting and auditing require little explanation to the EDP professional. The few differences between hospital business systems and those of any other commercial enterprise are straightforward both in concept and in implementation.

An idea that is receiving considerable favorable attention among hospitals with developed data-processing systems and competent staffs is the possibility of combining or integrating several of the discrete parts of a business system into

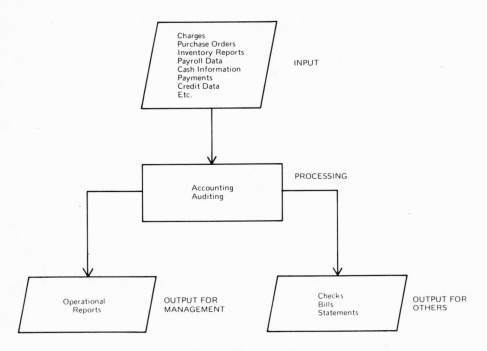

Figure 2.5   Data flow in the accounting area

one or more larger systems. Thus, payroll and personnel files might logically be combined; accounts receivable, payables, cash receipts, purchasing, and general ledger have so many interactions that an integration of the programs and files could allow for more efficient operation; and so forth. And of considerable value, the order processing data collected in the therapy system provide all the information needed for detailed patient charge assignment, thus reducing the amount of redundant data collection.

The other main area of innovation in hospital management data processing is in the development of appropriate forms, terminals, displays, readers, control units, and the like, for input/output in the many specialized areas of the hospital. Many of the I/O functions must be automated. Many others must not be automated. The selection of those areas where automation is appropriate and the designing of the proper type of automation are of major concern to the hospital EDP professional.

THE THERAPY SYSTEM

We may classify the therapy activities of the hospital, including what we have called diagnostic and rehabilitative functions, into direct and indirect patient care activities. Direct activities comprise all diagnostic and therapeutic procedures carried out by those people concerned with, and responsible for, the patient. These are, basically, doctors and nurses engaged in medical and surgical treatment of patients. The indirect activities are X-ray and laboratory tests, record keeping, admissions and discharge, and the like.

In an information systems sense, the vital activity of the therapy system, both direct and indirect, concerns patient data. All information relating to patient identification, history, treatment, diagnosis, test results, and the entire course of his illness are collected by some part of the therapy system. We may say that the entire input for this system is patient-oriented information.

It would be possible at this point to become quite specific and quite detailed concerning the types, formats, and quantity of patient-oriented data collected by the average community hospital during the average hospital stay. However, we will devote an entire chapter to this area later. Instead of considering specific details here, let us rather examine the progress of a patient through the therapy system, observing in a very general way at each stage or department the kinds of input, processing, and output that are currently useful or planned for the near future.

The first stop for any patient coming into the hospital is the admit desk. Here the basic data are collected concerning his complaint, the services to be given him, his insurance status or economic condition, and identification parameters. This information is compared with that of previous patients and with preadmission lists from staff doctors where appropriate. An account number is assigned to the patient and he is directed to a ward and bed. These basic data are used to build a skeletal medical record and start an accounting record for the patient. In addition, many hospitals order a series of standard blood and urine tests for all patients admitted unless the physician gives orders to the contrary.

On the ward, two kinds of information will be collected. The first of these is data concerning temperature, blood pressure, pulse, liquid intake, fluids excreted, and so forth—in other words, objective measurements of physiological functions. These data are taken periodically and recorded on the patient's chart, which becomes part of the medical record. The second type involves evaluation of observations and data, diagnostic comments, instructions for treatment, drug prescriptions, supply and test requisitions, and the like, which are collected from the doctors or nurses and forwarded to the appropriate service area. Most of this data also goes into the medical record. Since there is a continuing review of this activity by both doctors and nurses as they treat the many patients in their care, it is best to consider the medical record as both input and output for this part of the system. A patient's charts are consulted regularly by everyone concerned with his care.

The clinical laboratory receives test orders and samples from the wards, performs the indicated tests, and prepares reports on the test results for the physician and for inclusion in the medical record. In some cases, the specimen accompanies the test request; at other times, laboratory personnel are sent on rounds through the wards to collect or draw the specimens. A typical laboratory data flow diagram is shown in figure 2.6.

Information flow for the radiology department is very similar to that for the clinical laboratory. Input consists of physician requests for services to be performed, in this case, X-rays or radiation treatments; and output consists of patient schedules and test results. The internal processing is different in detail; but again from a data-processing point of view, not dissimilar. Some physical procedure is followed, in both cases, that leads to data concerning some aspect of the patient's body described in concrete terms. These must be evaluated and reported back to the patient's doctor.

The functions of the discharge area are quite simply to halt the process started regarding a patient at admission time and to close the medical and accounting records on that patient. Usually, this is not possible at the moment of discharge for several reasons. Many of the test and supply requisition cycles require more than one day for their completion. This means that some test results are not in when the patient leaves, nor are the charges for all services available at that time. On the other hand, few patients are willing or able to make total payment at discharge time, so that accounting must maintain an accounts receivable record on most discharged patients until the bill is paid. These factors are further complicated by the slow response in time by both government and private third party payers. The result of all this is that few, if any, records are truly closed at discharge time or even for several months

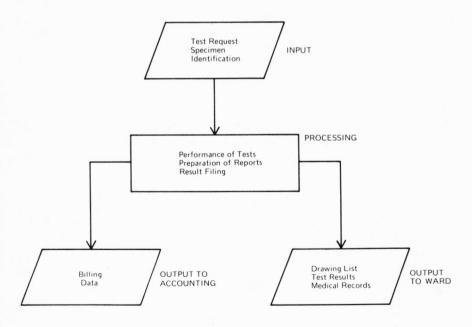

Figure 2.6   Data flow in the laboratory

thereafter. However, the inpatient side is closed, and the final procedures for closing all records are initiated at discharge.

We will now consider three of the almost unlimited applications of computers in the therapy system: computer-aided diagnostics, patient monitoring, and order processing. Books have been written on this topic, and the surface is just being scratched. The applications described below are proven, practical systems, not research projects.

There are two major branches to computer-aided diagnostics. One works from a patient history and questions asked through, say, a CRT terminal to arrive at a probable diagnosis or suggested possibilities according to built-in matrix tables presenting disease conditions versus symptoms and complaints. The other approach uses one or more physiological signals such as are given by the electrocardiogram or electroencephalogram as primary input, analyzes the signals by sophisticated mathematical techniques, and suggests a diagnosis on the basis of departure from norms of the signal. Of course, none of these applications attempt to dictate to the physician; they are aids to diagnosis and can make suggestions only. The final responsibility rests with the patient's doctor.

The monitoring applications are based on the recognized fact that patients with certain kinds of illness, such as coronary or pulmonary problems, and all patients who have been through major surgery are subject to cessation of respiration or organized heart activity. Many patients suffering acute respiratory or circulatory failure can be resuscitated if their condition is discovered in time. The time involved is often only a matter of seconds. Few hospitals have the staff to handle any significant number of patients of this kind by the method of continuous human vigilance. Thus the assistance of electronic devices to monitor certain physiological signals has become common.

The human body produces in its normal activity a variety of bioelectric, biomechanical, and biochemical signals, which can be detected by the appropriate sensing device and converted to an impulse readable by computer. At this point, the signal may be compared to the preset alarm conditions, and a light or buzzer will be activated if the signal is outside allowable limits. The value of computers in this area lies in their ability to monitor many patients with the same central unit, thereby allowing two or three nurses to handle eight or more patients.

During the course of treatment of a patient in the hospital, several service areas or departments in the hospital will be called upon to assist in his diagnosis or therapy by performing tests or supplying drugs, appliances, or other items. These items and services will be at the instruction of the attending physician, usually through the intermediary of the ward nurse. She will request a particular service by an order that must be delivered to the relevant service area, interpreted, filled, and returned to the nurse or doctor for delivery to the patient.

A data-processing system that is used in some variation in several hospitals operates in the following way to automate the processing of these orders:

1. A doctor order is input to the computer via an appropriately designed terminal at the nursing station.

2. This message is converted by the central processor into its parts, reformated for easier use by the service area, and transmitted to all interested hospital stations, including the service area itself, the business office, and medical records.

3. As the order is filled or as the service is scheduled or performed, the service area notifies the nursing station via its local terminal.

4. Editing and control features assure that a valid request is supplied and that all orders are filled as requested.

We shall see that the information concerning services performed can be used by many other application areas in the hospital. One of the most important of these is the patient's medical record.

THE COMMUNICATIONS SYSTEM

A very simple description of the function of the communications system is shown in the flow chart in figure 2.7.

In other words, data collected from any and all parts of the hospital are

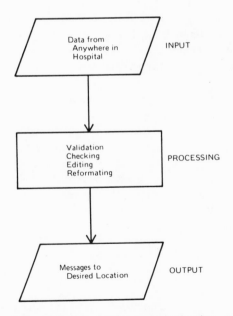

Figure 2.7   Data flow in the communications system

transferred to the desired location after being checked for accuracy. However, the communications system may be called upon to perform several complex tasks involving considerably more internal processing.

In the input area, it may be necessary to verify the authorization of the sender, the accuracy and completeness of the message sent, and the appropriateness of the desired receivers before an input item can be accepted. These factors are especially important in medication orders or changes for medical or accounting records.

Internal processing may be required for some of the checking and verification tests. A message log is a good management tool for measuring the effectiveness of the system and its utilization. Updating of records may involve editing and correction to preserve record quality, and a reformating of messages may be needed to conform to receiver requirements.

Output authorization is at least as vital as input authorization. Sometimes, as in an inquiry into a record, the two are the same, so that a check on both authorizations is necessary. Some messages require splitting so that one part will go to one receiver and other parts to another receiver. In some cases, a message may go to many receivers, in altered form for each.

Thus, it is obvious that the job of the communications system is an extremely sensitive one. It is not too much to say that the communications system is the nerve center of the hospital. Without appropriate information exchange, the hospital cannot function.

It should be obvious that most of the applications mentioned in the systems considered imply a very sophisticated communications system for moving information around the hospital. This system will have three main jobs. First, it must recognize the sending station, receiving station, and format of every message in the network, reformating where necessary and managing all switching activity. Secondly, it must assure the quality of the messages by various hardware checking and software editing modes. Finally, it must control the computer and communications hardware involved in performing the first two activities.

These functions suggest the use of a dedicated communications/file maintenance computer interacting with other machines in the hospital on demand. As the use of communications in medicine and in hospital operations grows, this dedicated system could absorb such tasks as closed-circuit television switching and control, maintenance and retrieval of all permanent data storage, control of automated bulk deliveries, and so forth. We will consider the design of such a system in a later chapter.

SUMMARY

We have attempted in this short introduction to provide the reader with some insights into hospital operation and into the kinds of problems the information-processing specialist will address. We have talked briefly about systems analysis, policy and planning, and information flow in the hospital. Many of these topics have been merely touched upon and will become subjects for more careful treatment in later chapters. Others such as hospital history, community health, and functional analysis are not considered central to our purposes.

In any event, we have met the subject of our study face to face. The hospital has been shown to be a complex social, physical, organizational, and functional entity, as well as a series of data-handling systems of tremendous variety. It should be obvious that this variety forms one of the major motivations for the introduction of automation technology.

For the next few chapters, we shall leave the computer behind us and concentrate on the functional aspects of the systems we have identified above.

REFERENCES

Hudenberg, Roy. *Planning the Community Hospital.* New York: McGraw-Hill Book Co., 1967.

Lindberg, Donald A. B. *The Computer and Medical Care.* Springfield, Ill.: Charles C Thomas, 1968.

Rosenfield, Isadore. *Hospital Architecture and Beyond.* New York: Van Nostrand Reinhold Co., 1969.

Souder, James J.; Clark, Welden E.; Elkind, Jerome I.; and Brown, Madison B. *Planning for Hospitals—A Systems Approach Using Computer-Aided Techniques.* Chicago: American Hospital Association, 1964.

3

The Service, Building, and Supply Systems

INTRODUCTION

While the three systems making up the title of this chapter are as vital as any other to the operation of the hospital, they have less involvement with our main area of interest, information processing, and are somewhat less instructive than the other three. Entire books can and have been written concerning small portions of the supply and environmental aspects of the hospital. The short sections that follow do not begin to do them justice, but they are amply represented for our purposes here.

THE SERVICE SYSTEM

The service system has been characterized in the previous chapter as having extremely limited requirements for information and correspondingly little effect on hospital data in general. Its functions involve the carrying out of basic clerical, maintenance, and janitorial duties, adding little to the store of information concerning either patients or hospital operation beyond the simple facts that certain tasks were performed. In stating this somewhat oversimplified picture, we must remember that we refer to the *service system*, an abstract, arbitrary division of functions in the hospital, rather than to the departments or their personnel involved in service tasks.

Thus, a ward clerk in her duties as unofficial nurse's aide may add materially to the observations about the patients on her ward. A clerk in the business office performs several vital functions—sorting, classifying, interviewing, and the like—of great importance to overall business data processing. Moreover, the maintenance engineer will often be responsible for the collection and retrieval of a whole variety of data concerning the hospital equipment and structure in his care. However, in performing these data-processing functions, the nurse's aide, clerk, and engineer are elements of systems other than the service system. Our purpose in dividing the hospital into systems by data-processing function has been to improve our understanding of the information-processing aspects of hospital operations. We must not lose sight of the fact that real hospital operation involves a great deal of repetition and duplication of duties and personnel.

We will consider four distinct areas in the service system: clerical, janitorial, maintenance, and special services. For each of these, we will describe briefly its activity and distinguishing features. For a more thorough treatment of any specific area, the reader may refer to the references at the end of this chapter.

Clerical Services

Clerical services include routine tasks such as typing, filing, transcribing, handling cash, unpacking, filling of nonpharmaceutical orders, shelving, admitting, and scheduling of appointments.

Owing to personnel or time constraints, much of this work is done by nursing or other professionals on the hospital staff; however, in some hospitals, special clerical personnel are becoming more prevalent. Ward clerks fall into this category. They are a relatively new addition to the hospital personnel complement. The motive for introducing special clerical help on the wards was to remove some of the paper-work load from the nursing staff, freeing them for more direct patient care. This work load approaches 40 percent of the average nurse's time in hospitals without ward clerks. The introduction of ward clerks has helped to reduce this figure, but lack of training, legal restrictions, and operational policies have combined to make the actual program less effective than it is potentially. In many cases, the appearance of the ward clerk has encouraged the transfer of some clerical duties from other areas such as the pharmacy or the clinical laboratory, thus partially defeating the purpose.

An area that traditionally has been staffed by clerical personnel is the business office. Most of the record keeping and handling of bills and payments are routine tasks assigned to clerks with minimal training in accounting. A similar kind of task is the admission interview, where basic insurance and credit data are taken from the patient or a relative.

The clerical duties involved in the purchasing and stores inventory functions of the hospital require more familiarization with the items and procedures common to health care facilities. At the very least, a working knowledge of medical terminology is essential. Many hospitals carry on a continuous program of orientation for new personnel, especially where the turnover is high. A few institutions have borrowed a good idea from industry and are providing employee training and enrichment programs leading to supervision.

Janitorial Services

All cleaning activities, whether of the hospital's interior or of the exterior building and grounds, are classified as janitorial services. In addition to the obvious regular cleaning, special prompt attention must be paid to the preparation of patient beds as soon as they are vacated. It is essential that incoming patients have these beds as quickly as possible. In most hospitals, admission and discharge times are scheduled so that the housekeeping division has adequate time to change linen, vacuum, sterilize and restock the room before the new patient arrives.

Care of external grounds includes landscape maintenance, gardening and grooming, window and exterior cleaning, and care of parking lots and other open areas. The importance of these tasks to the general appearance and operating efficiency of the hospital cannot be overestimated.

Maintenance Services

One of the eternal verities of life is that everything becomes worn out, used up, or broken. It is the job of the hospital maintenance services to repair or replace the structural, mechanical, and electrical portions of our impermanent hospital world. These services have, in general, two aspects, a preventive maintenance program and an on-demand or emergency repair function.

Preventive maintenance is of extreme importance in a hospital. Lives often depend upon the functioning of critical equipment such as motors, lights, pumps, and electronic sensors. To insure reliability in this vital equipment and in the other costly and delicate devices in the hospital, the maintenance staff inspects them on a regular, rigid schedule, oiling, lubricating, repairing where necessary, and replacing doubtful parts or those subject to failure, even if no damage or wear is evident.

Most good-sized hospitals have facilities for the repair of furniture, small machinery, and electrical appliances. In a large hospital, the machine, electrical, and carpentry shop may rival any industrial maintenance shop. With adequate staffing and good management, the modern hospital can be relatively independent in these areas, calling on outside help only for major reconstruction or replacement.

For certain specific equipment, particularly complex electronic devices such as X-ray machines, laboratory instruments, and computer hardware, the hospital depends on maintenance contracts with the manufacturer or a service company.

Special Services

A few service activities in the hospital do not fall under the usual classification scheme. These include the chaplaincy, the various auxiliaries, and voluntary groups and social service. Their work is vital to the goals of the hospital, both from a public relations aspect and as a matter of good medical procedure. The American Hospital Association recognizes that these activities are a necessary part of total patient care and recommends that qualified staff and adequate facilities be provided, as well as the support and cooperation of the administration and other hospital personnel. The hospital is encouraged to participate in the formation and implementation of effective programs in these areas and to formulate policies that will tend to foster their growth.

THE BUILDING SYSTEM

The complexity of modern buildings, especially in their mechanical and electrical systems, has increased in recent years for even the smallest buildings. Air conditioning, temperature, humidity, pressure, power and heating, and all the myriad motors, fans, relays, pumps, boilers, indicators, gauges, and meters that must be read, started, stopped, or adjusted several times daily, make automation of some kind a necessity. Likewise, protection of property and personnel by automated security and disaster control equipment is sound management.

It is probably fair to say that no other kind of building needs and deserves the comfort and protection of automated systems more than the modern community hospital. There have been few published studies to support the belief that building automation directly improves patient care. However, industrial climate control has been shown to increase personnel productivity, decrease costly mistakes, and, in general, add to the morale of the work force.

There is little question that the expensive equipment housed in the hospital requires protection from fire and smoke damage, vandalism, and theft. In addition, the special problems of the hospital in evacuating the critically ill demand special treatment that can be given only by automated systems. The reasons, then, for automating the hospital building control systems are many, both economic and humanitarian. Let us examine the major areas of building control—environment, security, and disaster—to discover what these systems do and how automation has been applied.

Environmental Control

The usual building control systems for air conditioning, temperature, and humidity are, of course, present in the hospital. In addition, some areas require more stringent control of these parameters as well as of others unknown in most buildings. Examples are: (1) laminar airflow in operating rooms, wherein sterile air passes over the table and personnel in one direction only, cutting down the chances of airborne infection during surgery and (2) special control of dust, water vapor, and combustible gases wherever static electricity could be a problem.

The many special environmental demands for specific kinds of illness as ordered by the professional staff must be met by the environmental control system. These include temperatures above or below normal, high or low humidity, and enriched oxygen atmosphere. Moreover, they must be provided to special areas without interference with normal hospital ambient conditions.

These requirements imply control over several hundred widely dispersed points in the building, involving examination of parameters; checking against desired operating conditions; adjustment, starting, or stopping of equipment; and integration of all points into a total picture of building conditions. For the building engineer and his personnel to make the rounds of these points several times daily would be impossibly expensive and probably ineffective. Thus, at the very least, some central point is needed from which all equipment and systems can be monitored and controlled.

Once the data from the building are collected, they must be analyzed before appropriate action can be taken. Analysis here means comparison with normal or desired values, computation of usage and efficiency, tentative decision on action needed, and investigation of the effect of proposed action on other system parameters before it is taken. Centralization of measurement and control solves part of the problem, but the complexity of the computation and interaction procedures and the response times required in many hospital situations indicate that much more extensive use of automation is advisable.

Automated building systems for hospitals have been a reality for several years. Their response to hospital problems has taken fairly standard forms. These systems permit the programming of most of the building's operating functions without the intervention or attention of engineering personnel. Central scanning or alarm sensors in real time allows immediate response by maintenance personnel; and most of the computation and analysis of building performance, including the logging of important information, can be done by computer. Automated systems control building operation where human intervention is unnecessary and provide data for decisions where the building engineer requires personal control.

Security Control

Building security systems are classified according to alarm location, type of installation protected, and type of danger protected against. Alarms are commonly placed in three places: the immediate area of protection; a central control point for the entire building; or the offices of police, private guard, or other protective agency. It is characteristic of security systems, as opposed to other building automation, that very little action is taken beyond the notification of responsible persons that intrusion or compromise has occurred.

Three types of facility or installation protection are commercially available: perimeter protection alarms on intrusion at any point of entry on the boundary of the area protected; area protection alarms on the presence of unauthorized persons within a given area (for example, motion within a room after hours would trigger an alarm); and object protection alarms on disturbance of a single object such as a desk, safe, or cabinet. This means that it is possible to provide protection against an intruder at three separate stages—his point of entry, the area through which he must move, and the object whose security must be assured.

The usual security system is designed to protect against burglary or theft; however, access control to sensitive areas is another valid application. For example, the operating suite during surgery must be protected from infection by unsterilized personnel or equipment. Similarly, contagious or critically ill patients, as well as highly susceptible newborn babies, must be isolated from unauthorized personnel and visitors. Security systems offer protection from all these dangers.

Disaster Control

Disaster in the ordinary office building usually means fire. That is the case in the hospital also; yet disaster may occur in other forms, such as smoke, explosion, noxious or combustible gases, sudden power loss, and so forth. The hospital disaster control system must be designed to respond to any of these quickly and reliably with the appropriate alarm or countermeasure. When the lives of bedridden and critically ill patients are at stake, the time required to evacuate, isolate, or otherwise protect must be shortened by every means possible.

Fire alarm systems have been in common usage for many years and have proved themselves in countless potentially fatal situations in hospitals. Two kinds of action are automated in the typical system. First and foremost, the hospital personnel must be warned of the fire hazard. Detection sensors for fires include high temperature and temperature gradient sensors, smoke or combustion product detectors, and infrared radiation sensors. Alarms may be of the sort that warns all within hearing or may be keyed to warn hospital personnel only. The alarm may be audible or may consist of flashing lights or may combine both. In some cases, direct connection to a local fire department warns the fire-fighting agency automatically. It has been shown that the early warning of emergency conditions coupled with practiced fire safety procedures are the best preventive measure against loss of life and property by fire.

The second action, usually automated, involves some kind of positive countermeasure. The building system is capable of providing a degree of protection against fire loss by the automatic water sprinkler, carbon dioxide, or other extinguishing material. These methods are especially useful in supply and storage areas where few personnel and no patients are located. Medical records or film storage, central supply, receiving docks, and the pharmacy are good examples.

Another common function of a fire control system is to partition the hospital into small areas with fireproof doors, thus isolating the fire and restricting its ability to spread to unaffected areas. In some storage areas, these doors may be closed automatically upon detection of a fire hazard. For the rest of the hospital, operation of the fire doors must be manual to avoid danger to personnel and patients.

Many of the methods used for smoke detection will also detect the common toxic, combustible, or explosive gases that might be present in a hospital. The important responses here are to inform responsible personnel and to clear the air as quickly as possible. It may be necessary to isolate a storage area if a gas cylinder ruptures.

Explosions are a danger in hospitals, especially in surgery, where many of the common anesthetics are explosive in high concentrations. Use of anesthetics and the attendant risk of explosion must be included in the plans for a disaster control system. There is a trend away from the use of these anesthetics; but as long as they are used, the hospital must be prepared to cope with the possible consequences of their use. Of course, the best protection is to utilize procedures that will insure that gas leakage is kept within acceptable limits. When these procedures fail, early detection of the leak before explosive concentrations are reached can minimize the danger. If an explosion does occur, there is danger of related fire along with injuries and damage to life-sustaining equipment. It is vital that blastproof fixtures and power terminals be used in the hospital wherever there is danger of explosion.

THE SUPPLY SYSTEM

The provision of the enormous quantity and variety of medical and clerical supplies required by the community hospital is one of its most urgent needs. There are literally thousands of items in the hospital supply catalog. Proper management of this difficult function demands detailed and timely information concerning all aspects of the supplies and their consumption.

There are three basic problems associated with supply administration—inventory management, order processing, and delivery control. In addition to these factors common to any supply application, there are special hospital considerations, such as sterile processing and packing, drug supply, and narcotics control. We shall treat some of these special problems in their specific area of application; but before we discuss the special problems of hospital supply, a few words are in order concerning the more general factors mentioned above.

Inventory is a stock of various supply items kept on hand to provide a service to users, to feed a production line, to provide goods for sale on demand, or to keep vital activities operating, while waiting for further deliveries. Inadequate inventory has immediate harmful effects in work stoppage, unfilled orders, or dissatisfied customers. On the other hand, excessive stocks create problems of capital reduction, spoilage, storage costs, obsolescence, and the like. An unbalanced inventory, in which some items are overstocked while others are chronically short, results in the worst of both worlds.

The problem of inventory management is to maintain for each stock item a stock level and a replenishment schedule such that demand during the delivery interval is just met by the stock on hand. Of course, many difficulties and complications are ignored by this simple view. Since much of the replenishment mechanism is outside the control of the supply department, a safety stock is kept on hand to protect against faulty or late deliveries. Many vendors give quantity discounts, special prices on sale items, and total cash discounts, all of which will vary from time to time. Demand is subject to random, seasonal, or periodic variations for some items. For these and other reasons, it is not possible to set stable stock levels and reorder schedules in most real supply situations. Dynamic adjustments are necessary to minimize costs while maintaining service. The adjustments depend upon several factors. The computations and procedures are beyond our scope of interest, but a brief discussion may be helpful.

The first step in dynamic inventory control is the forecasting of the demand for the items in stock. If we know the demand with accuracy, we can plan stock levels to meet that demand. We can never have that knowledge, but there are techniques for estimating future demand based on past consumption and for giving confidence levels to those estimates.

On the basis of these data, we can specify when a stock item will reach its danger point and thus should be reordered. The next question is how much to order. The answer to this question depends upon many factors in addition to demand. Several formulas have been developed for estimating what is called the "economic order quantity" using the various costs involved in placing an order, storing the items, unit costs including discounts, administrative costs, and so forth. These formulas suffer from a common difficulty in obtaining accurate cost figures, but their use has proved of value in real situations in spite of the theoretical problems.

The above calculations must be done for each item of inventory. Then the many interrelationships must be investigated. Because of vendor quantity discounts on some items and total order discounts for large orders, as well as the cash and special sale prices, the unit cost of an item may vary from period to period, and even within the same period, depending on the order mix. These calculations can become extremely complex and time-consuming. They are prohibitively so for manual inventory control systems, and even for computer processing there is a point at which further computation becomes more costly than the possible savings in unit cost.

Whether a manual or automated system is used, it is clear that none of the calculations are meaningful without accurate and timely data on inventory parameters and vendor activity. An audit of stores and an update of vendor information must be a continuing feature of an inventory management system.

There are several methods for notifying the various supply areas of an institution that an operating unit needs a particular item from stores. The most common method involves the use of a document called a *requisition,* which is the written form of an *order.* The handling of these documents is called *order processing.* Order processing in the usual supply department, warehouse, or company stores consists of five major steps:

1. Verification of items, quantities, and dates requested and of the authorization or credit rating of the requestor

2. Checking of order against inventory for outages or substitutions

3. In case of outage, checking with requestor for substitution approval or back order instructions

4. Issuance of picking lists and packing slips to stores clerks

5. Preparation of order for delivery, notification of accounting, and simultaneous updating of inventory records.

The most serious flaw in the above set of procedures is the possibility of time lags between steps 4 and 5. When this lag occurs, an order for an item may reduce inventory to zero, but another order for that item will have gone through step 2 before the inventory records are corrected. This causes much delay in processing the second order, which may encourage the resubmission of the order, thus confusing things still further. A reduction of this time lag is very difficult in a manual system.

The delivery of orders once they are filled and packed has many aspects in an industrial environment that are not of great interest to us here. Such matters as scheduling of delivery vehicles, freight rate structures, en route spoilage, economic order groupings, packing fractions, and the like, are of little importance in a hospital setting as hospitals are operated currently. However, as we shall see in the next section, there are delivery problems of great complexity peculiar to hospitals.

We will particularize the above comments for four specific supply areas in the hospital: bulk stores, food stores, central supply, and the pharmacy.

Bulk Stores

Bulk stores in this book include all the items used by the various hospital departments with the exception of food items and pharmaceutical supplies. The pharmacy and the kitchen have special storage and preparation problems requiring separate treatment. Certain items pass through a sterilizing and prepackaging process before distribution, and others are recycled through the sterile area after use. These will also be treated in a separate section.

Pricing and volume considerations dictate that most of the items purchased by the hospital will be in bulk, that is, in case, carton, barrel, or other large quantity lots. Unpacking, shelving, and sorting these supplies into storage areas are dusty jobs, usually kept separate physically from the clean supply areas, such as linen storage or surgical supplies. It is estimated that a hospital will need 30 to 40 square feet of storage area per erected bed. This is a sizable investment in space alone; so that the methods mentioned above for minimizing space requirements are attractive. However, service to users in a medical environment demands, that certain goods be available on request without fail. This may be a matter of life and death in some instances. Economic considerations cannot be given an overriding voice in such decisions. A control system must be devised to insure maximum service on selected items while providing needed control on other supplies.

One of the major considerations in the design of the stores control system is the kind of delivery system used by the hospital. Two major alternatives are in common use, the requisition method and the complement method. In the requisition method, each item released from stores must appear on a requisition form signed by an authorized person, such as a nurse, a doctor, or a supervisor. This method is often defeated by the practice of releasing goods on telephone authority, accepting the promise of a requisition that seldom materializes. The items are delivered to the requesting department on regular messenger rounds or by pneumatic tube or dumbwaiter, or they may be picked up at stores in case of urgent need.

The complement method utilizes carts or cabinets left in the area of use, stocked with a large percentage of the items needed at that station in quantities sufficient for most situations. The carts are restored to full capacity at regular intervals. An inventory count is kept at the central department so that usage can be distributed over all departments, but requisitions are needed only if an item not found on the car is required. Both these methods have their advantages and disadvantages, and both are in wide use.

Rapid automated delivery systems using conveyor belts and electronically guided carts are bringing about a merging of the requisition and complement systems. A request keyed in at the nurse's station can trigger the automated filling and delivery of an order for most of the items used in the hospital. By keeping track of usage, the nurse can inform the inventory computer how much has been used of each item on her cart at the end of her shift. These data can be used to restock the cart, also using the automated order filling and delivery system. There still remain questions concerning the necessity of this degree of automation and its cost with respect to the current methods.

Dietary Stores

Because food processing management is more qualified to judge the condition of perishable or damaged foodstuffs than the usual receiving clerk, special purchasing and receiving areas and personnel are provided in the dietary department.

Storage bins, walk-in coolers, and freezer compartments are required equipment for dietary receiving, as well as a large amount of dry storage space for canned and packaged goods.

The dietary department should be designed so that there is a smooth flow of materials from receiving, through storage, to processing and preparation, to central distributing, and up to the patient's bedside. In addition, adequate provision must be made for the return of recyclable dishes and utensils and for the disposal of waste products. Some of the parameters that affect the design of the dietary department are: the number of beds, type of general supplies distribution, amount of preprocessed and precooked food used, type and number of special diets, degree of patient freedom in menu selection, and so forth.

One of the basic elements of hospital food processing is the planning of the menu. There are several entree choices on the standard daily menu and also dozens of special diets, such as low calorie, high protein, low sodium, low bulk, liquid, ulcer, diabetic, and so forth. The dietitian must plan a total hospital menu containing an attractive and tasty combination of dishes for the ordinary patient; for those with special requirements; and for the staff, personnel, and visitors who eat in the cafeteria. Since the patient load varies both in number and type of patient, the menu must be dynamic, flexible, and responsive to the hospital census.

Once a menu plan is adopted, it must be broken down into its constituent foodstuffs. A net requirements purchasing list is made up from these data and available inventory reports. The ordering and delivery of items are planned to coincide with preparation time requirements. Menu plans generally cover 30-day intervals.

It should be obvious that no simple manual system could do this set of jobs economically. The usual solution is to keep a very large inventory to insure service, as in other hospital supply areas. However, spoilage and other losses are extremely high for food storage, and experience has shown that this method leads to repetitive and uninteresting meals, a common complaint of hospital patients. There could be no more natural candidate for inventory management techniques than the dietary department. Furthermore, in the meal planning area itself, some significant savings in time can be made by linear programming methods applied to the problem of nutritional adequacy constrained by dietary restrictions.

Sterile Supply

The services performed by this division of the supply system consist of provision, sterilization, dispensing, and recycling of practically all supplies specifically oriented toward medical or surgical patient activities. Not all supplies from this area are truly sterile, but a sufficient proportion is of this nature to make the entire department a clean area with much more severe storage requirements and processing conditions.

Processing generally refers to the collection of soiled items, their sorting into groups and categories, inspection for damage or special cleaning problems, and the washing and sterilization of all reusable items. The sterilization is done by dry heat, steam, ethylene dioxide gas, or some combination of these methods. It consists of replacing the air in and around the item to be sterilized with the sterilizing medium, thus killing any bacterial or viral matter not removed by the washing. For some items an antiseptic soaking for a period of a few hours is sufficient. After the articles are sterilized, they are packaged under sterile conditions in treatment trays, surgical packs, or other convenient forms for reuse. A plastic film or cellophane wrapping may be used to maintain sterility in storage.

As in food processing, the flow of items from cleaning and sorting, through sterilization, and into packaging and storage must be smooth and foolproof. Sorting and cleaning work areas must be physically separated from sterilization areas, and the latter should be protected by alarms to insure against the compromise of sterile conditions.

In most hospitals, the central sterile supply service makes use of the same distribution system as the other supply departments. New advances in disposable treatment supplies and paper surgical "linens" have simplified many of the processing problems of sterile supply. Of course, sterile storage and careful handling is still of the utmost importance.

The Pharmacy

The functions of the modern hospital pharmacy are many times more complex than in the past. In addition to the traditional dispensing of drugs and solutions and the managerial duties associated with quality control, supplies, and equipment, the pharmacist has become an important member of the health care delivery team. He must be aware of the total range of medical care provided by his hospital and the interactions of the drugs he dispenses with other aspects of patient care.

We may classify the tasks of the pharmacy as manufacturing, dispensing, and record maintenance. We will ignore the purchasing and inventory activities, since they do not differ materially from those of other hospital supply areas. It should be mentioned in passing that, traditionally, hospital pharmacies have acted independently in the purchasing and inventory functions. This is not unreasonable, since the storage areas are separate and the vendors normally not common to the other hospital supply departments.

Two methods of dispensing drugs are common in the hospital, the bulk system and the unit dose system. In the bulk system, medications are purchased in large quantities—bottles of several hundred grams of loose powder, liquid, or tablets. Prescriptions are filled by manufacturing capsules in the hospital or by pouring tablets from bulk bottles into individual paper cups for distribution to patients. Often, for nonnarcotic drugs, the nursing station will order 100 tablets for a patient, to be given over several days; and the nurse will make up each individual dose. Many difficulties are evident in this method, especially in control of dosage, loss of leftover medications, and further loading of the overworked ward personnel. The unit dose system was designed to solve some of these problems.

The advent of unit dose distribution has reduced greatly the amount of preparation and manufacturing of prescribed drugs for the hospital inpatient. (Outpatient pharmacy activities are relatively unaffected by unit dose systems.) This new method of dispensing drugs starts with a supply from the manufacturer that is packaged in individually wrapped doses in sterile packages, the sizes of which depend on the particular drugs and the usually prescribed amounts. Some drugs come in tablet, capsule, or liquid form, and so on through the more than 7,000 items in the possible hospital formulary. A request for a given drug can be filled in most cases by selecting the appropriate number of unit doses of the prepackaged drug. Most hospitals still elect to do some manufacturing, especially of rarely used items and parenteral solutions. But the immense amount of labor and the uncertainty of quality and inventory control have been reduced significantly in those hospitals using the unit dose system.

Reports indicate mixed feelings on the part of pharmacists, doctors, and nurses concerning unit dose; but there seems to be little doubt that it is here to stay. Changes in the storage and distribution methods and in record-keeping procedures must be instituted along with the unit dose system to take full advantage of its potential value.

The dispensing of drugs according to the doctor's prescription is the traditional function of the pharmacy, and certainly this function has lost none of its importance in modern hospital pharmacy practice. More and more diseases are treated at some stage by chemotherapy. It has been estimated that every hospital patient receives between two and three prescriptions on the average each day he is in the hospital. Other responsibilities, however, are becoming of equal importance to dispensing drugs; the hospital pharmacist is becoming a clinical pharmacologist. The major force behind this change is the increasing size and complexity of the pharmaceutical inventory and the growing concern about drug incompatabilities.

This term refers to the impact of certain drugs and drug combinations upon the condition of a particular patient. Incompatability may take five basic forms: (1) sensitivity or allergy to a given drug or class of drugs, (2) interference of a drug with some other prescribed or patent medication, (3) interference between a drug and certain foods, (4) contraindication of a drug in a specific clinical situation, and (5) interference of a drug with certain laboratory or other diagnostic tests. These are areas of traditional responsibility for the physician, but there is a growing attitude among pharmacists that the complexity of modern drug therapy makes it impractical for the physician to keep abreast of developments in this area along with the rest of his work load. Thus, the pharmacist, as the only professional qualified to do so, must take upon himself some of the responsibility for assuring that the drugs he dispenses do not fall into one of the above classes of incompatibility.

Clearly, the pharmacist must have a great deal of information concerning both the drugs he dispenses and the patients for whom they are intended if he is to discharge adequately the new responsibilities of clinical pharmacy. Data on such matters as diagnosis, condition, treatment and surgical procedures, diet, and so forth, are vital to an evaluation of the patient's drug regimen. A glance at the record-keeping functions of a hospital using unit dose methods indicates the magnitude of the information-processing problem. The following are typical steps in dispensing drugs to a new patient:

1. The name, location, and record number of a newly admitted patient are forwarded to the pharmacy. Similarly, any change in location must be given also.

2. A drawer for medications is assigned in the pharmacy; and another, on the patient's ward. Often these are drawers in medication carts.

3. A *drug administration document* is started. Each prescription is recorded here, including drug name, dosage, form, frequency, times, and check boxes for actual administration.

4. These entries are triggered by a *physician's order form,* filled in by the patient's doctor and sent to the pharmacy.

5. The pharmacist checks the order for correctness and incompatibilities by comparing this order with the patient's *medical profile form* and his *drug administration document.*

6. The drugs ordered for that ward for the entire coming shift are made up and placed in their appropriate drawers for delivery. These are entered on a *cart checklist* for verification by ward personnel.

7. If for any reason a drug is not given at the indicated time, a *drugs-not-given notice* must be filled in at the ward.

8. Narcotic orders are usually stopped within 48 hours of prescription automatically. A *notice of automatic stop* order is made out and sent to the ward by the pharmacy.

The purpose of all these forms and procedures is to provide the information needed for effective control of pharmacy functions and to maintain checks and audit trails for each instance of administration of a drug to a patient. It is basic that every medication should be recorded and that every patient's medical record should have a drug profile showing every medication received while in the hospital.

REFERENCES

U.S. Department of Health, Education, and Welfare. *General Standards of Construction and Equipment for Hospital and Medical Facilities.* Public Health Service, Publication No. 930-A-7. Washington, D.C.

Gorham, William R. *Business Office Activity Analysis.* Hospital Systems Improvement Program. Ann Arbor: University of Michigan Press, 1968.

Hudenberg, Roy. *Planning the Community Hospital.* New York: McGraw-Hill Book Co., 1967.

McGiboney, John R. *Principles of Hospital Administration.* New York: G. P. Putnam's Sons, 1969.

Messerschmidt, Mary L. *A Study of Central Service Distribution Systems at the University of Kansas Medical Center.* San Antonio: Baylor University Press, 1969.

Soltis, Steve J. "Mobile Supply Closets Save Time, Money." *Journal of Hospital Management,* vol. 93, no. 5 (May 1962).

Zook, M. Lorraine. *Disaster Plans.* Washington, D. C.: The George Washington University Press, 1966.

4

The Management System—
Part I: Fiscal Management

INTRODUCTION

The management system has been divided into two logical structures, fiscal management and policy making. It must be remembered that this division is arbitrary. There is a great deal of information exchange and commonality of personnel and procedures between the parts; however, there are enough differences in the details of their operation and their areas of responsibility to make separate treatment useful from a data-processing viewpoint.

Fiscal management is a varied and difficult topic, encompassing fund-raising, financial planning, accounting, auditing, budgeting, and investment planning. The relevance of many of these topics to data processing in the hospital is questionable. In this chapter we shall focus our attention on those areas that affect or are affected by data processing in a direct fashion.

It is virtually impossible to understand the workings of any large organization without some familiarization with its fiscal procedures. Every business, institution, and government agency has financial aspects, expenses, income or sources of funding, bills to pay, salaries and wages, taxes, and the like; these monetary aspects are expressed in the language of accounting. As we study hospital operations, we find that many of its problems are expressed in accounting terms. Accounts receivable, patient billing, cost allocation, third-party reimbursements, and internal auditing form a partial list of these areas of interest.

In addition to being of general interest to anyone studying hospital procedures, they are of especially vital interest to the hospitals' data-processing personnel. In a sense, fiscal management can be considered a specialized branch of information processing. The aim of accounting, to provide data to management for decision making, is a data-processing aim; and the methods of accounting—the record keeping, the summarizing, the evaluation—all these are classical data-processing methods.

It should come as no great surprise that fiscal systems are the first application of data processing in most hospitals. The problems of a financial nature are the most pressing and the most easily recognized by the typical board of trustees. Moreover, the methods of attack, the electronic accounting systems, are straightforward in application and easily judged in performance, compared to the more exotic biomedical computing systems.

The accounting function is not necessarily a bad choice for entry into hospital computer usage. A good accounting system collects information on virtually every transaction, both medical and financial, that occurs in the hospital and also on the operation of every functional area. With this data on hand, many purposes may be served beyond the narrow needs of the business office. Thus, the usage of the computer in the hospital tends to grow outward from its starting point into other areas of application.

In the present chapter we shall examine some of the features of accounting, especially as it is used in a hospital environment. Note that it is not our purpose to train accountants. This overview will not treat any accounting system in detail, nor will extensive background for any accounting functions or procedures be provided. General principles will be stressed, a few concepts perhaps new to EDP people will be introduced, and some accounting terminology will be explained in terms more familiar to the data-processing professional. The aim is to make hospital accounting problems and methods more understandable, so that the applications in these important areas become more meaningful. The explanations given are from a data-processing viewpoint, not from an accounting viewpoint.

The fiscal systems to be treated will be given the generic name *accounting*. This term may not be strictly accurate, but a most common usage among hospital business data-processing departments is to classify their activities as hospital accounting. That usage will be followed in this text.

In order to focus our attention, we may turn to figure 4.1, which illustrates the typical divisions of a business office and some of the more common transactions flowing among them.

THREE ASPECTS OF ACCOUNTING

We may view accounting functions as having three basic aspects: past activity, ongoing activity, and future activity. These do not correspond to actual procedural differences. In fact, every accounting procedure may be looked upon

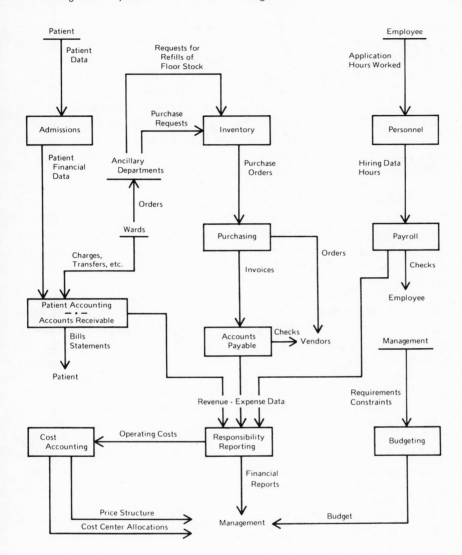

Figure 4.1   The hospital business office

from all three viewpoints. But the emphasis of the analyses and the use made of the results may be clarified by a chronological classification.

Current activities are of two kinds, record keeping and transmittals. The various ledgers, journals, registers, files, inventory records, and so forth, are created in the course of the daily activity of a business. These records become a permanent documentation of performance and the basis for all accounting analysis. We shall look at these in more detail in later sections. Transmittals are action-oriented documents directing disbursement of funds, requesting purchase or payment, or otherwise dictating some financial action. When the action has been initiated, the transmittal becomes a part of the record of that transaction. Together these two types of document form the data handled by the accounting department in relation to its ongoing day-to-day activity.

The accountant looks at past activities to evaluate performance during a given fiscal period. As we shall see, he may also wish assistance in formulating plans for the future. Evaluation of past activities involves an analysis of costs and accomplishments and also a comparison with expected values. Evaluations of this kind are termed *cost accounting* and *auditing*. We will spend some time on each of these as they pertain to hospitals.

Future activities may best be illustrated by the well-known financial planning procedure called *budgeting*. This involves an analysis of such past activity as may be helpful in estimating future costs, trends in income and expenses, setting of rates charged for services—in short, all the data needed for generating a plan for hospital operations based on financial constraints. Hospital budgets are an important part of the information-handling task.

These distinctions may be clarified by viewing them in a more computer-oriented manner. Consider the accounting activities in the hospital as being real-time, delayed-time (batch), or forecast/simulation jobs in a multiprocessing/multiprogramming job stream. The processors are the various individuals and subdepartments of the business office involved in the multitude of accounting tasks. Since the division of labor is seldom complete, each subdepartment may have several tasks. Thus, the cashier will handle payments to patient accounts and at the same time be updating other accounts. The accounting department is a true multiprocessing/multiprogramming environment.

Real-time tasks in the job stream are those requiring immediate attention. Incoming charge and payment data must be captured, or they will be lost. This is similar to an analog-to-digital sampling with a random sample rate. The important thing is to record the data as they are being acquired. How to process the data, what they mean, and so forth, are decisions to be made later.

Similarly, requests for payment should be given immediate response in order to preserve the reputation and credit rating of the hospital and maintain employee morale. This is very much like an interrupt-driven communications processor, which must acknowledge a request from a terminal upon receipt of an interrupt on that line.

These real-time tasks are just the ones mentioned under the heading *current activities*. The temporal references *current* and *real time* do not imply any specific response time. They are merely convenient terms to designate a difference in mode of operation triggered by different accounting needs. We may think of record keeping as a kind of data acquisition and sampling task and of transmittals as interrupt acknowledgments without compromising our understanding of the real nature of hospital accounting. On the contrary, this may help those of us with differing backgrounds to reach a commonality of terminology more quickly.

Delayed-time or batch jobs are those that may (or perhaps must) operate in a background partition: they do not require immediate attention, or perhaps they require data not available to the foreground. This corresponds to data reduction tasks performed on data collected in real time, but processed in a batch mode. This is an adequate analogue to the auditing function. Cost accounting can be thought of as yet another mode of reducing the same basic data. It is in this sense, the nonreal-time sense, that we talk of "past activities."

Forecasting is a special kind of batch job in which data are produced that may be used to control some of the machinery involved in the real-time data-acquisition tasks. This is the closed-loop feedback type of system that utilizes data collected and processed to predict future events and then varies the control to alter those events in specific ways. No better description could be found for the entire budgetary process than a "future activity."

The above paragraphs indicate the possibility of a model that would view the hospital as a physical system with various processes in motion at various points in the system. Accounting would appear to be a sensor/control system, acquiring data through random sampling techniques by several foreground processors; analyzing the data in several batch modes; and producing, among other things, a set of control parameters that are fed back to the original system.

We shall not carry this model any further in the text, but it shows promise as a means of studying some of the processes involved in hospital accounting. Its importance to us here is to point out the way in which our unorthodox terminology is to be understood. If the accounting procedures are clearer because of it, the terminology has served its purpose.

CURRENT OR REAL-TIME ACTIVITIES

We have divided current activities into records and transmittals for purposes of discussion. It should be emphasized that these are really different views of the same transaction. As a transaction is initiated, a document specifying further action is generated. As the action proceeds, the documents become records. Without records of prior transactions, there would be no way to determine the kind of transmittal needed today; and without transmittals, there would be an incomplete record of today's transactions. Let us look, then, at several common transactions in several accounting functions to see what transmittals are used and what records are generated.

Payroll

The purpose of the payroll function is to record work performed, compute compensation due, pay appropriate funds, and record funds paid. In addition, such side benefits as sick leave, vacation, insurance, and the like, must be recorded as earned and used; and certain city, state, and federal deductions must be recorded, accounted for in the employee's check, and paid to the proper government agency. Procedural information flow is found in figure 4.2.

1. A new employee fills out various hospital and government forms detailing dependents, optional deductions, and other pertinent information.

2. These data, along with hospital-provided hourly rates, shifts to be worked, vacation and sick pay schedules, and so forth, are recorded in a master personnel file.

3. Hours worked and the station or department are recorded on an employee time card on a daily basis. They are submitted on a regular schedule to the business office.

4. The time cards and the data from the employee master file are used to compute earnings, taxes, and other information for the given pay period; and a check for the net amount is printed and released to the employee.

5. On a monthly basis, a report is generated to inform the general accounting area of funds paid out during that month.

6. On a quarterly basis, tax and insurance deductions are accumulated; and checks are sent to the appropriate payees.

In this and the functions that follow, we have skipped over many of the complications and difficulties in the actual procedures; but the general flow of information and the kinds of records and transmittals generated should be clear.

Accounts Payable

Accounts payable procedures are designed to keep records of creditors, make payments, record purchases and receipt of goods, and maintain accurate records of all transactions. Control is the key. Costly mistakes and fraudulent manipulations occur more frequently in the accounts payable area than in any other function. Typical control procedures are:

1. Assume the purchasing department, at the direction of one of the operating cost centers, has ordered certain items from a vendor. In the course of the vendor's accounting activity, a document called an *invoice* will be generated and sent to the hospital. This document forms the fundamental payables transmittal and constitutes a request for payment. In it are itemized the kind, quantity, and price of each item ordered; the discount applicable; the terms (30 days, on receipt of goods, and so forth); and the total amount due.

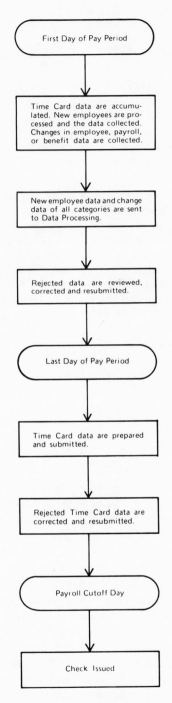

First Day of Pay Period

Time Card data are accumulated. New employees are processed and the data collected. Changes in employee, payroll, or benefit data are collected.

New employee data and change data of all categories are sent to Data Processing.

Rejected data are reviewed, corrected and resubmitted.

Last Day of Pay Period

Time Card data are prepared and submitted.

Rejected Time Card data are corrected and resubmitted.

Payroll Cutoff Day

Check Issued

Figure 4.2   The payroll function

2.   As soon as the purchased goods are received, inspected for completeness and breakage, and approved, a memo to this effect is sent to the accounting department. The memo is compared with the original purchase order and the vendor invoice.

3.   If no discrepancies are found, a voucher is issued, causing a check to be sent to the vendor. If for any reason the goods-received memo does not match the invoice and the purchase order, a series of exchanges with the vendor takes place until agreement is reached upon a correct invoice amount, at which time a check voucher is issued.

4.   Occasionally, shipping errors are discovered, and goods are returned after the check voucher has been issued. In this case, a document called a *debit memo* is sent to the vendor, explaining the circumstances. A copy is also sent to the hospital business office. When the appropriate credit memo is received from the vendor, the ordering departments are credited with the returned amount, the previous voucher is canceled, and a new voucher is issued in the correct amount. Much of the data vital to this activity relates to vendors, their addresses, discounts offered, minimum quantities, and so forth. This information is maintained as part of the routine accounting activity.

The *voucher system,* as the above set of procedures is called, fits very well into the needs of hospitals for responsibility reporting, that is, the assignment of expenditures to the responsible departments. It is somewhat cumbersome, but its control and verification features outweigh its disadvantages for many voluntary hospitals.

Accounts Receivable

The most complicated accounting function performed in the hospital involves accounts receivable. For most businesses, the accounts receivable function has five basic ingredients: the recording of services rendered and amounts charged; the preparation of bills and recording of collections; the classification of payments and maintenance of balances for individual and departmental accounts; the analysis of account balances, preparation of statements, and organization of receivables by the length of time nonzero balances are outstanding (aging); and reporting periodically for general accounting purposes.

The motive for all this activity is to maintain control of business income. Hospital accounts receivable have the same ingredients; but they are much more complex because of the differences in inpatient and outpatient procedures, third-party billing, professional services, and the huge volume and variety of charges to each account. The following steps have been simplified for an easier grasp of fundamentals, though the vital factors are included. We shall discuss some of the complicating factors in a later section.

1.   As a patient is admitted to the hospital as an inpatient or arrives for his first visit as an outpatient, an accounting record is initiated; and certain identifying data and insurance coverage information are taken.

2. Charge slips detailing services rendered to the patient are collected and posted to his account daily. These charges are of three basic types: room and board and general nursing care; professional services and supplies; extras and luxury items. Amounts for these charges are posted by the accounting department and based on established rates unless a special price is stated on the charge slip.

3. For patients without insurance, an itemized bill covering all expenses is sent shortly after discharge. For patients with insurance or who are covered by a government health program, a proration of charges covered and charges payable by the patient must be performed before the first bill is sent out.

4. Payments from both third parties and the patients are posted daily as received. The entries form part of the daily journal.

5. An aged accounts receivable report is prepared monthly. At the same time, statements of amounts owed are sent to nonzero balance accounts.

6. An income performance report by department is prepared for general accounting every month.

Records and Transmittals

We have discussed several kinds of transmittals (payroll tax deduction forms, payroll check vouchers, invoices, purchasing vouchers, and debit and credit memos) and several kinds of records (employee master files, check registers, vendor lists, general accounting reports, patient charge slips, and daily journals) used in the ongoing financial activity of a hospital. These documents interact to provide hospital management with information and control over financial affairs. Since good records produce transmittals and since transmittals always become part of the record, the distinction between them is artificial. The emphasis on control is the important point. All the complicated forms and procedures are designed to insure control. If authorized transmittals are insisted upon for every transaction, responsibility is always clearly delineated; and if every transaction is recorded, errors are minimized. That is the purpose of accounting.

PAST OR DELAYED-TIME ACTIVITIES

The review of past fiscal performance in a hospital is required both by law and by good business practice. Performance can be measured in two important accounting modes. One involves a careful study of the accounting procedures, control operations, and detailed handling of financial affairs by all members of the hospital personnel complement. This is called *internal auditing,* and it functions by evaluating the effectiveness of the control system. The other mode attempts to develop and control the costs of services, supplies, and operations within the hospital. This is called *cost accounting* and functions by analyzing the relationship between expenditures and departmental output. Both of these activities aid hospital management in meeting its responsibility for carrying out its goals efficiently and economically.

Cost Accounting

In determining costs for any business, we must take three steps. First, we must measure the expenditures applicable to income performance during a given accounting period. Then we must relate the derived costs to the measured output of each department or general ledger cost center. Lastly, both of these steps must be considered in the light of the purpose of the analysis—whether it is recommending changes in business operations, proof of requirement for larger facilities, or a study of the operating efficiency of a given department manager.

For the voluntary hospital, the major purpose of its cost accounting procedures is to insure that all expenses incurred in its operation are covered by the charges to users. In other words, each department must charge a rate for its services and supplies that allows it to cover its cost of operation. Measuring departmental expenditures is simplified by assuming that each department is a small independent business, buying from other hospital departments or from outside; collecting its own income; and sharing equitably in the common costs of plant, utilities, clerical services, and the like, with the other departments. A unit cost is derived for each item sold, and this is charged to whoever uses the item, whether patient or other department. Output is measured in terms of services rendered and charged. Thus, even nonpaying patients or professional courtesy allowances are charged at the established rates insofar as accounting is concerned.

The problems with this method of cost accounting are many. Allocating and distributing costs to the various departments are not straightforward tasks. Establishing unit costs for services is difficult. Moreover, the effort involved in this analysis is immense. Still, third-party contractors and even state law in some areas require these cost figures for reimbursement and control.

Internal Auditing

Auditing in a hospital serves much the same function as in any other business. This is the provision to management of an objective appraisal of hospital financial procedures along with detailed recommendations for improvement where needed. To be effective, the appraisal must be a continuing activity closely associated with systems and procedures or operations research, though with more emphasis on accounting procedures.

Internal audits are called for by the administrator or the board of trustees, and the audit report is submitted to the board for approval and action. The report is based on exception; that is, reports are made upon only those aspects of the hospital that contain errors or discrepancies, factual but unwarranted situations, weaknesses in control procedures, inefficiencies, or any other functional problems.

The breadth and scope of auditing are reflected in the data reviewed by the internal auditing department. All financial data are, of course, examined and checked, as well as operational data from all departments. In addition, the auditor will interest himself in any and all activities that seem to him to be significant to the hospital's well-being or to which he is directed by his management.

FUTURE OR SIMULATION ACTIVITIES

A budget is a plan for the future operations of a business over some specified period expressed in accounting terms. Three kinds of budget are common in the hospital. The *operating budget* is an estimate or forecast of expenditures and income for the coming fiscal period. This is usually a composite and compromise made up of individual departmental budgets. The *capital budget* is of much longer duration, five to ten years or longer, and relates to building, plant, expensive equipment, and other large expenditures. Most hospitals also utilize a *cash budget* to insure that enough cash is on hand to cover expenses and to take advantage of cash discounts, but that excess cash is invested to produce income.

The creation of a financial plan is only one part of the budgeting activity. Close supervision of all personnel is required to insure that the budget is being used as a guide to their efforts. It should be remembered that budgets are plans based on estimates. If the estimates are in error or if unexpected events occur, there must be enough flexibility in management to account for this and to change the budget. Changes must be accompanied by justification, but we must never refrain from beneficial activities, nor should we continue with ineffective activities, just because the budget so states.

Thus, evaluation of performance as time passes is an important part of the budgetary process. The purpose of planning is to provide management with criteria for measuring how well the organization is meeting its financial goals. Monthly ledger reports should be examined in terms of those goals; and appropriate steps should be taken, either by changes in personnel or procedures or by changes in the budget, to bring practice into agreement with theory. It should be noted that monthly changes in budget indicate poor budget preparation, whereas excessive procedural modification or personnel turnover may reflect poor administrative control. Healthy flexibility is not the same as uncontrolled change. Management treads a thin line between concrete and spaghetti.

Two kinds of data are vital to the budget function: past activity and performance, including previous budgets, and predicted future needs and events. The performance of the hospital is available from the reports and statements of the previous years. Forecasts are more difficult to obtain and much less accurate.

Continuing activities can be predicted with fair precision from last year's figures and some estimates of growth rate. New activities and allowances for the unexpected can only be guessed. Examination of experiences from similar institutions and consultations with experts can be helpful, but in the final analysis only second- or third-year budgets of a new activity have any hope of accuracy.

THE ACCOUNTING PLAN

The methods and procedures used by an organization in recording, classifying, summarizing, and reporting financial data are characteristic of that organization. The accounting plan used by most voluntary hospitals is compatible with the *Uniform Chart of Accounts* of the American Hospital Association (AHA). The main features of the accounting plan are: fund accounting, accrual basis for income and expenses, account classification uniformity, rate assignment, and compatibility between manual and machine methods. Let us examine each of these features briefly.

Fund Accounting

A fund is a division of resources or liabilities by means of accounting procedures, allowing the separate reckoning of certain aspects of a business. A hospital divides its resources into several funds, partly for convenience and partly because of legal restrictions on the use of some assets. For example, a large donor may stipulate that his gift may be used only for X-ray equipment. This would require a separate fund to be set up to manage his gift, unless an X-ray fund were already in existence.

Hospital funds commonly in use are the general operating fund, the permanent endowment fund, the plant fund, and the collective investment fund, each of which has its own usage and restrictions. In addition, the system usually leaves available several temporary funds that may be utilized for various short-term purposes.

Accrual Basis

Accrual is a term used by accountants to indicate a particular method of recording income and expenses. There are two fundamental aspects:

1. All income is assigned to the period in which the services involved in earning the income took place. In the nonaccrual basis, income is recorded as it is actually collected.

2. All expenses, supplies, labor, professional services, rentals, and so forth, are charged to the period in which they were used or consumed. This is opposed to the nonaccrual procedure of assigning costs to the period in which funds are expended, items purchased, or services contracted. In addition to the above features, the accrual basis includes depreciation as an operating expense rather than as a separate item.

Account Classification

The analysis of income and expenses into an accurate picture of operating performance on a monthly basis is one of the responsibilities of the accounting department. This job is rendered much easier by the adoption of a numerical coding of income and expense items to be used by all departments and cost centers in the hospital. There are several schemes in existence, and any of them can do the job. Since there is some value to the ability to compare similar performance figures between hospitals, a standard used by most hospitals in the United States was adopted by the American Hospital Association. A manual entitled *Uniform Chart of Accounts* describes this system.

Rate Assignment

One of the activities of the accounting department described in a previous section, "Cost Accounting," had as one of its goals the derivation of a unit cost for all items of supply or service in the hospital. Once a rate has been established based on these unit costs, the expenses of the providing department will be covered if the volume has been forecast with reasonable accuracy. This procedure allows positive control over departmental expenditures and avoids complex monthly allocations. When a uniform accounts chart is maintained, types of service are easily identified and compared. Quarterly rate adjustments, along with some retroactive interdepartmental fund transfers should be sufficient to keep the hospital departments within the budget.

Compatibility

The accounts classification system is given a numerical coding to make automated or machine accounting procedures more feasible. The forms and procedures used by most voluntary hospitals and recommended by the AHA are applicable in a manual, mechanical, or electronic environment. It is of utmost importance in this, as in all medical data-processing applications, that the procedures utilizing automated equipment be compatible with some kind of manual system. No machine failure may be allowed to interrupt the prompt and effective control of hospital activities.

THIRD-PARTY CONTRACTS

An aspect of hospital affairs not found in the usual business is the relationship of the hospital to third-party payers. These include Blue Cross and other health or hospitalization insurance companies, Medicare, and the various state and local government agencies involved in guaranteeing health care. We shall see in the next chapter that the effects on hospital policy of the account of third-party activity are very significant. These effects are even more striking on hospital financial affairs.

In recent years the proportion of hospital charges paid by parties other than the patient and his family has increased dramatically. The growth of health service contractors has many interesting social and economic aspects, but per-haps the most relevant to our purposes is their effect on hospital accounting procedures. In this sense, they all have similar requirements. These requirements involve immense amounts of clerical and auditing activity in order to qualify for reimbursement. Furthermore, since costs are not uniform among hospitals, each one must repeat the same basic steps individually.

When we consider the variations in labor costs, transportation fees, and general economic conditions across the country, it is easy to see why compre-hensive cost figures and uniform charges for services are impossible for American hospitals. Because of this lack of uniformity and because of the substantial variability in the relation of costs to charges, most contractors have instituted a cost reimbursement method for calculating payments to participating hospitals. By this method, a per diem cost is determined for each hospital by dividing total allowable operational expenses by total patient days in the operating period. This would seem fair if all operating costs were allowed, but the exceptions are many and expensive. Usually, the rates are set based on the previous operating period, with some retroactive adjustments based on actual expenses.

Allowable costs specifically exclude all hospital activities collateral with, but not directly involved with, patient care. Some of these activities are research, teaching, and charitable works. Another area of large expense to hospitals involves bad debts. Many hospitals feel that bad debts are part of the normal operating expenses of a hospital, but third-party contractors uniformly do not allow these as reimbursable cost items. Some interest and depreciation items are allowed, but under strict limits.

One additional way of controlling costs is practiced by many contractors. This is the variation of per diem cost with occupancy level. The theory is that the hospital must be encouraged to operate at optimum occupancy levels to maintain a proper balance between patient care and the economic advantages of large-scale operation. An occupancy of between 80 and 90 percent is considered optimum. This allows for high utilization of facilities and full staffing, yet leaves room for emergency conditions. At about 70 percent, contractors are of the opinion that some of the per diem cost represents unnecessary facilities; and a percentage of the per diem cost is discounted. These figures will vary somewhat with special conditions such as new hospital facilities, prevailing economic conditions, and location. Some amount of negotiation on these matters is possible. Another factor providing some cost-conscious incentives to hospitals is the variation of reimbursement rates with average length of stay. The total cost to the contractor is a function of the number of admissions and the average cost per admission.

SUMMARY

There are many similarities between hospital accounting and its counterpart in an industrial firm. Its purpose is much the same, the control of income and operating costs so that the goals of the organization may be achieved efficiently and economically. A hospital represents a large aggregate of capital, as does an industrial facility. Its income is derived from services rendered, as in most businesses. Moreover, administrative efficiency is as much a measure of performance in a hospital as in a factory.

But there are many differences too. Most hospitals operate on a nonprofit basis. Their operating costs do not, as a matter of ethics, include advertising; and the goals of the institution are directed outward toward their patients rather than inward toward stockholders or owners. Accounting in a hospital setting is one of the methods of control utilized to insure that financial affairs continue to serve and further those goals.

The accounting procedures outlined above are designed to assist hospital personnel in maintaining the day-to-day and long-range control of hospital finances. By providing management with information and analyses needed to form intelligent decisions, accounting plays a vital role in the operation of the modern hospital.

REFERENCES

American Hospital Association, 1957. *Cost Finding for Hospitals*. Chicago.

Seawell, L. Vann, *Introduction to Hospital Accounting*. Chicago: Hospital Financial Management Association, 1971.

Taylor, Philip J., and Nelson, Benjamin O. *Management Accounting for Hospitals*. Philadelphia: W. B. Saunders Co., 1964.

5

The Management System – Part II: Hospital Policy Making

GOALS AND POLICY

No more vital activity to the healthy functioning of a hospital can be found than that set of operations directed toward defining institutional goals and specifying means for achieving them. The result is a plan of action, hopefully conforming to prudence and efficiency, called *policy*. The policy-making process reviews the aims and motivation of the hospital, sets priorities among them, determines requirements for successful implementation, and, most importantly, allocates available resources according to the specified priorities.

The data-processing specialist will seldom be called upon to judge hospital policy or to contribute to its formation; however, a knowledge of the mechanisms and people involved will be of value in designing data-processing applications. The goals of the EDP department will be more easily realized if a weather eye is kept on policy changes.

One of the most striking aspects of the policy-making process is change. Every hospital grows and changes under the stresses of internal and external pressures. Influential people leave or enter the organization. Legal or regulatory restrictions are imposed or modified. Funding sources are discovered or depleted. Public opinion becomes more or less favorable. In addition, all of these may require significant changes in policy to insure optimum operation. Opinions and goals of policy makers also change, and policy may be modified at times to follow idle whim.

In this chapter we shall examine in some detail the factors that tend to cause significant changes in hospital strategy; the process by which these factors are taken into account; and the people who are involved, officially and unofficially, in the policy-making process in a relatively important way.

As an example of policy making, we shall examine the question of data processing. Assume that a hospital with no internal data processing has been asked by a vendor to consider the purchase or lease of a computer. The accounting functions have become more extensive than the current manual system can handle, and many areas in the clinical departments have been pressing for computers also. We should like to know the internal and external considerations affecting this policy decision, the way various groups in the hospital are involved in the decision, and the process by which the decision is reached.

POLICY

The administrative complex found in the modern hospital has characteristics encountered in few environments, either industrial or institutional. The organization, the informal hierarchy of status and influence, the multiple formal and informal channels of more or less dependable communication—all tend to complicate an already difficult task, that of managing an institution that must be run by businesslike processes toward an unbusinesslike goal. A business, furthermore, the customers of which purchase services they would rather not have and the quality of which they are unable to judge.

These factors and the many others affecting hospital strategy are a source of problems to policy makers. For purposes of discussion, we may categorize these factors as part of the external environment, considerations of institutional resources, effects of internal social groupings, or actions of important individuals.

External Environment

The effects of the outside world on the hospital fall into two convenient classes. Restrictions or constraints placed on some aspect of hospital operation by a governmental agency, a professional or labor organization, or a community group expressing public opinion make up the first class. These may be economic constraints, conditions of licensure or accreditation, contractual obligations to employees, terms of acceptance by the medical staff, and so forth.

Basic legal standards for licensure are established by the authorized state agencies with the guidance of medical advisory councils. These must be adhered to by any institution operating as a hospital in that state. The advent of Medicare has imposed additional regulations upon participating institutions.

These include acceptable cost accounting methods, minimum service standards, and a multitude of mandatory forms and reports.

Most governmentally imposed standards are stated as minimum acceptable requirements. A hospital aspiring to excellence will need to go far beyond these minimum standards. To encourage objective measurement of patient care quality, the American College of Surgeons, an association of physicians in all areas of surgery, initiated in 1917 a program directly concerned with surgery in hospitals. The standards developed by this organization were used nationwide for more than 30 years. As the scope of the program grew and the number of involved hospitals increased, it became necessary to broaden the base of support of this activity to include other organizations. In 1952 the Joint Commission on Accreditation of Hospitals was formed, with representation by the American College of Surgeons, the American College of Physicians, the American Hospital Association, and the American Medical Association.

Over the years, the standards have been elaborated, extended, and improved as medical knowledge and practice have changed. Though no hospital is required by law to attain accreditation, the Joint Commission supplies one of the most prestigious and effective ways of demonstrating the quality of services offered. The hospitals are very few that do not have or aspire to have Joint Commission accreditation.

In addition to the above, hospitals have felt pressure from insurance carriers, nurses, clerical and maintenance unions, financial organizations, and suppliers of hospital goods. Virtually every area of hospital operation must meet some kind of externally imposed code or be subject to legal sanctions, loss of prestige, or public harassment.

In the typical community hospital, many of the above effects are operative. Part of the reason for the heavy load on the accounting system is the increase in reporting requirements imposed by government agencies and insurance carriers. This may be the most important single reason for the automation of hospital business functions. In addition, the reports of university hospitals and the various medically oriented journals have created an atmosphere of expectation in the minds of physicians of more effective patient care methods based on computers.

The second class of external effects concerns changes in facility utilization owing to increased demands for services, natural disasters, accidents, or civil disturbances. An urgent need has developed for standby medical facilities, which can be called upon and staffed by emergency personnel, in the event of a requirement for hospital services beyond the ordinary capacity of community hospitals to deliver.

Hospitals are expected to do everything possible to plan and prepare for emergencies, but sometimes planning is inadequate, and even advance notice is insufficient. For example, since medical care for social security recipients has been discussed since the Truman Administration, this should have provided some advance notice to hospitals of impending increases in demands for services; yet when the 1965 amendments to the Federal Social Security Act, which set up a program of health insurance for the aged (Medicare), became effective on July 1, 1966, no one was ready.

Many people covered by this law were financially able for the first time in their lives to obtain adequate medical care. Years of deprivation had augmented the debilitating illness connected with aging, so that the care required was often of an urgent nature. In addition, without the restraint of lack of funds, many people requested and received treatment for minor conditions that would have been ignored before the existence of Medicare. The overall result was a flooding of health care facilities far beyond expectations. Funding provided under medicare has not allowed hospitals to keep up with this huge increase in the demand for services.

This extreme overcrowding of the patient care areas of the hospital has produced a parallel increase in the clerical load in the business office. This increase has pushed many hospitals toward computerization in order to be able to handle the huge accounts receivable volumes. Another motivation has been the fund shortage. It has been hoped that automation will prove to be more economical than manual methods or that capture of lost charges and greater productivity will present a better cost picture.

The kind of services offered by hospitals has been changed in recent years in response to public demand. Sophisticated diagnostic and therapeutic equipment and procedures have been added because medical practice required them, but an acceptance of the changing role of hospitals in society has encouraged the extension of hospital activities into social services, public health education, and home health care. The increased awareness of the social responsibility of hospitals has come about largely because of external pressures.

Institutional Resources

Possibly the most pervasive problems of hospital policy are in the area of resource allocation. The problems usually resolve themselves into selecting among competing needs for the provision of inadequate or, at best, scarce resources.

Funding is the most obvious and perhaps the most inadequate resource in the hospital. Building costs may run as high as $35,000 per bed, while annual operating costs may reach $12,000 per bed. The total cost of services, personnel, and facilities approaches $20 billion nationally in the 1970's. Barring radical changes in the organization and delivery of patient care services, we can expect these costs to increase with our expanding economy.

Health care personnel are an equally vital resource of the hospital. The Health Services and Mental Health Administration of the United States Public Health Service estimates that almost four million persons work in some 375 professions and occupations related to health care.

The investment in the physical plant must be considered an important hospital resource. This figure is currently about $30 billion, covering buildings and capital equipment in about 7,500 hospitals across the country. Allocating space within a hospital to the conflicting special interest groups, the medical departments, wards, laboratories, and ancillary services, is a major area of concern to hospital management.

An important resource too often ignored is public sentiment. In the final analysis, all hospital resources, funds and personnel, come from society at large either through taxation, direct fees, and indirect payments by insurance carriers or through donations in fund-raising drives. Thus, it is obvious that a positive image is conducive to a better-endowed, better-staffed, and better-utilized hospital. Too often, good publicity in the major media is considered sufficient. There is, however, a growing realization that public opinion is molded by every employee, staff member, trustee, patient, and area of the building and grounds and that rumor can be as powerful as fact. As in politics, the appearance is as important as the reality. Public relations in the Madison Avenue sense is an important part of image building. But there is no PR substitute for sound and sympathetic patient care; understanding attention to social and financial problems; and a clean, cheery atmosphere in the wards, halls, and grounds of the hospital.

Resource allocation studies are also of importance in deciding whether to utilize a computer or not. Estimates of manual costs displaced by a computer performing the basic accounting functions run from $3.00 to $7.00 per patient day. These assume enough manual effort to duplicate the reporting capabilities of a computer, an unreasonable effort for most hospitals. On the other hand, this reporting effort may be required for reimbursement in the near future.

Since the 1930s, hospital admission rates and outpatient visits have doubled, whereas the ratio of hospital beds and physicians to population has remained almost constant. Clearly, the demand for services has far exceeded the supply. This leaves an allocation problem of horrendous proportions for hospital management.

Social Systems

The goals of an organization can be achieved only by the cooperative action of individuals. These individuals may or may not share these goals, and the sharing of common goals may be less important than the sharing of activities. Still, in the broad medical field, it is considered vital to encourage an attitude of dedication and devotion to patient care and to inspire feelings of loyalty toward the hospital.

The extent to which this is possible is dependent to a large degree on the smaller groupings of individuals within the large organizational units. These groups may be official entities such as medical staff committees or personnel labor unions, endowed with authority and recognized by hospital management. When this is the case, there is an accepted mechanism by which their views may be expressed and their influence legitimized; but often the more influential of these groups are informal, voluntary associations, unnamed, unrecognized, sometimes *sub rosa*. They cut across departmental boundaries, ignore official barriers, and develop communication lines often more efficient than trustworthy.

In any event, wise hospital management will be aware of the existence and importance of these groups and be prepared to elicit their support or cope with their opposition. Often, a knowledge of the lobbying and bargaining for position among the several groups in a hospital will be of more significance in understanding policy formation than a study of organization chart models of administration.

Individual Behavior

In any organization there are individuals who stand out as leaders by virtue of their ability to influence group choices. Often, these qualities are recognized by the official structure, thereby creating an effective institutional officer, department head, or supervisor. Almost as often in hospitals, this is not the case; and other less official means are employed by the individual in the exercise of his leadership. These means may or may not tend to be disruptive of hospital procedures or counterproductive in relation to hospital goals.

It is vital that the effect of these individuals on hospital strategy be properly recognized and assessed. Policy decisions are choices among several alternatives. The methods by which the selections are made and the motivation behind them are the results of the character and behavior of individuals.

POLICY MAKERS

The above comments may have seemed to stress the role of the administration in coping with the problems of our health care delivery system. Actually, the administrator is one of a team of hospital officers faced with this task. Every hospital worker is concerned with, and has effect on, policy to some degree. It should be clear that policy must be implemented to be effective. Some of the people that implement the policy and thus influence its effectiveness are the same people responsible for its formation. This is in sharp contrast to the usual industry or corporate policy board, which is isolated from line authority, at least in theory. We shall see that the ambivalence created by conflicts in interest and professional goals forms a unique challenge to those involved in hospital policy making.

Three groups stand out, at least in an official sense, as having clear-cut responsibilities and functional distinctions: the governing board, the administration, and the medical staff. It is helpful to examine each of these groups and their functions separately before attempting to define their relationships.

The Governing Board

As a preamble to our discussion, a reminder is in order concerning the kinds of hospitals under examination. Federal institutions are excluded since the board of governors for these hospitals is the Congress of the United States. Many state and county hospitals are operated under executive order, with the board (when one exists) having only nominal status. We also exclude proprietary hospitals, those operated for profit, because many of the conclusions drawn from examining these few small institutions could not be generalized safely to apply to other kinds of hospitals. Similar considerations exclude hospitals run by religious bodies. The remaining hospitals, commonly referred to as *community hospitals*— the nonprofit, nongovernmental, community-owned, and community-sponsored hospitals—make up about 40 percent of the nation's hospitals and comprise some 25 percent of all assets, expenses, and personnel.

Data-processing usage in hospitals varies with the type of ownership. Virtually all federal, state, and county hospitals have on-site computers and qualified data-processing staffs. Hospital chains, whether religious or proprietary, are rather well penetrated also. The community hospital has not been a good market for computer vendors to date for reasons to be discussed later. This fact presents a problem to the person who suggests the leasing or purchase of a computer to the management of a community hospital.

In the following paragraphs we shall examine the composition of the boards of the subject hospitals, the nature and extent of their authority, and the ways in which they discharge their responsibility.

There are more than 50,000 members of boards of community hospitals across the country. The number of trustees in hospitals varies from seven to several hundred. The titles also vary, with governor, trustee, and director being the most common. Although the Joint Commission on Accreditation recommends no specific number or title, it does outline in its requirements that the board hold regular working meetings; that written minutes, bylaws, and procedures be kept; and that committees be appointed and charged with specific duties.

Men who sit on hospital boards are usually prominent members of the business and professional community. Often, they are large financial contributors or have donated time or service to hospital fund-raising drives. Occasionally, broad community representation is sought either on a geographic basis or by seeking board members from the financial, labor, religious, and citizens' action groups in the community. More often than not, individuals are chosen on the basis of social prominence, though there is a recent trend toward recognition of the knowledge and skills needed for effective participation in the governance of a modern medical facility. New members are chosen by a nominating committee, and the choices are ratified by the full board at an appropriate membership meeting. The Joint Commission and also state law in most states require that the procedures for nominating and electing board members be included in the bylaws; however, the basis for selection and the qualifications used are left to the individual hospital's discretion.

Typically, factors that influence the selection of members are poorly defined. There is no more important policy in the hospital than that of choosing board members; yet the process of selection is too often given only cursory treatment by hospital policy makers, who are frequently pressed by urgent demands. Many researchers have called for more careful thought with regard to the problem of setting criteria for board membership based on some objective view of the job requirements and the desired results. As yet, little action can be seen in this direction. Instead, men reach the board with little understanding of what their function is or how they got there and with no assurance that they are qualified to carry out the tasks they have undertaken.

The board of governors is charged with the ultimate responsibility for all financial and operational aspects of the hospital. The board must decide questions of organization and personnel, provision of funds and their allocation, budgets and planning, professional standards, criteria for the acceptance of staff physicians, quality of patient care, and enforcement of businesslike, efficient management of the hospital's resources. This set of tasks can be gathered under the basic goal of providing the highest quality care to hospital patients within the resource capabilities of the institution. However, defining and measuring the quality of patient care is not a simple matter. As we shall see, the above goal is valuable as a statement of the central function and charter of the hospital, but careful and extensive research is needed to refine a knowledge of area health facility requirements, to quantify community willingness and ability to provide funding, and to specify the portion of service to which a given hospital should address itself.

A statement of responsibility is meaningless without an accompanying statement describing the group, agency, or individual to whom one is accountable. In the case of governing boards in community hospitals, one does need to look far for immediate accountability. Most of the voluntary hospitals were built for the people in the community with donations provided by these people. In a legal sense, every corporation, profit or nonprofit, exists with the express consent of the electorate. It is implied in this consent, for the hospital corporation at any rate, that inefficient operation or lack of responsiveness to community needs could result in the removal of consent through one of the legislative, judicial, or regulatory agencies, and a replacement of the governing board by some other administrative mechanism. In practice, the professional associations, the Joint Commission, and community pressures tend to keep virtually all boards operating in a fairly responsive and conscientious fashion.

A major difficulty encountered by the board in its policy deliberations is the measurement of the community. How does one determine the health needs and desires of the "people in the community"? Who are these "people"? What is the geographic and demographic nature of the area of service? If need and desire for health services and facilities conflict, how does policy resolve the differences? Wrestling with these questions has left many board members with ambivalent feelings concerning their understanding of the health care delivery system and its administration. Although there is mounting concern from within and criticism from without that hospitals are not well managed, the objective indicators do not support the majority of complaints; most boards are functioning well in most areas, but seem themselves to be unsure of it. Many conflicts and tensions are created in the hospital by these doubts. The hospital wishing accreditation by the Joint Commission must show that its board is an effective governing body for the hospital; that its constitution, bylaws, and procedures are explicit and followed; that its members evidence interest and concern by committee activities and regular attendance at board meetings; and that there are cooperative working arrangements among the various operating departments of the hospital. These requirements are exactly what any good board of governors will wish to fill in order to manage the hospital well.

We shall see that the ambivalent attitudes of the board affect data-processing policy as well as other hospital policy, though in different ways. The board is torn between its desire to conserve hospital funds and its natural inclination toward business data processing. The resolution of this dilemma depends to a large degree upon the strength of the medical staff and the wisdom of the administrator.

The Administrator

One of the duties of the governing board is to appoint as its representative the chief executive officer of the hospital, usually called the administrator. Though he is officially an employee of the board, we shall see that his influence on policy matters exceeds this nominally subordinate status.

Administration traditionally has been thought of as the implementation of specified institutional action to achieve the goals set by policy. This endeavor follows the same basic principles of good management no matter what institution is being managed. These principles may be enumerated as follows:

1. Analysis and evaluation of conditions
2. Formation of policies, goals, and means
3. Effective organization of resources
4. Application of resources and means to achievement of goals
5. Continuing evaluation of results.

The problems to be analyzed are presented by the interaction of hospital operations and external events with the goals set by institutional policy. In connection with meeting these goals, the specification of concrete objectives is one of the most important functions of administration. Interpretation of overall policy and the fragmentation of goals into manageable tasks for the various departments are necessary preliminaries to policy implementation. As objectives are laid out and assigned, continuing evaluation of resources and their utilization must be made. Management by objectives implies that objectives will be clearly and explicitly specified, that means for achieving them will be supplied, and that measures of effectiveness and success will be derived. These are all functions of administration.

The modern hospital administrator is a recognized professional, the only hospital officer with the training and inclination to attain a comprehensive view of all financial and technical aspects of hospital operations. As the representative of the board, he is expected to interpret board policy and intentions to his department managers and the medical staff. On the other hand, as the only lay individual with expert knowledge of the demands of quality patient care, he must be prepared to inform and advise board members on clinical matters, often supporting the medical staff in their quest for better methods and equipment, augmented capacity, or expanded services.

His position, however, has not always been so highly regarded. The hospital was a much less complex institution up to about 1940. Its problems were simpler. The practice of medicine and thus the methods of hospital patient care were changing very slowly. External events had much less impact. Resources were relatively plentiful; yet third-party sources and the restrictions they bring were limited. The administrator was called *superintendent*, and his job was basically custodial. He was definitely not part of the policy-making team. He reported problems with equipment and building facilities and presented bills and expenses for payment authorization by the board. He often was asked to wait in the foyer while policy matters were discussed.

The advent of the scientific practice of medicine has been responsible for a great many changes in the treatment of the ill and injured, not only in the specifics of clinical care but also in the administrative structure needed to supply and maintain the necessary hospital resources. As problems have increased in number and complexity, the training required to understand and cope with them has also increased. By the end of World War II, the title of the chief executive officer had changed to *administrator*, and his relationship to institutional strategy had changed from a passive to an active role. Much of his time was spent with funding sources, governmental agencies, third-party carriers, Joint Commission representatives, and so forth, rather than in the day-to-day operation of the hospital. The administrator in most modern hospitals may be closely compared to the executive vice-president of a commercial firm. It has been recognized generally that formal education in hospital management or public health administration is an important, if not indispensable, preparation for managing today's hospitals.

The job of the administrator is not purely technical. It is as much dependent on his knowledge of personal relationships as on his knowledge of accounting or public hygiene. His position is a very influential one and can be extremely potent in policy considerations if he is astute in handling the special interests and conflicting forces in his hospital. There is, however, a basic paradox related to the policy team in the hospital. The legally responsible body is the board of trustees. Since they hold the purse strings, they are the policy makers. The business of a hospital is medical care, and the doctor is the only one who has the knowledge and the permission to practice medicine. Therefore, he must determine policy in the hospital. The only full-time professional in the hospital with the broad educational background, the experience, and the organizational status to view all phases of the hospital in proper perspective is the administrator. Therefore, he should decide policy matters.

Being unable or unwilling to resolve this paradox, most community hospitals continue to operate like a headless beast with three legs. This has produced an uneasy state of truce between the warring factions. It is within this seething, amorphous struggle that the administrator must work to bring order out of chaos. This is, of course, somewhat exaggerated for dramatic effect. Hospitals do operate, and rather well, when one considers their problems and the scarcity of resources to solve them. Still, students of management tend to throw up their hands at the thought of an organization so totally outside the scope of management theory.

It is within this atmosphere that the administrator must consider whether or not to recommend computerization. Usually, the size of commitment of funds required to automate hospital functions is one that can be made only by the board of directors. Thus, the job of the administrator is advisory. However, this job can be very persuasive; in fact, determinative. It is essential to win the support of the administrator if the data-processing decision is to be a favorable one.

One of the unique features of administration in a hospital as compared to its counterpart in industry or government is the fact that the medical staff, the professional group most deeply involved in the main business of the institution, does not work directly for the institution. The medical staff, with the exception of the interns and residents, operate outside the authority of the chief executive. They are paid by the patient or his insurance carrier and negotiate with the patient independently of hospital control. We shall have much more to say in the next section concerning the medical staff. The important consideration at this juncture is that the doctor is a guest in the hospital and that treating patients in the hospital is a privilege he enjoys because of his staff membership. He uses hospital equipment and supplies, admits and discharges his patients, and directs hospital personnel in all matters pertaining to their care; but he is under no supervisory control by hospital personnel.

The hospital administrator must manage an organization devoted to providing a service to an unwilling customer, and he is without legal control over the funding and other resources essential to that service and without authority over the personnel most closely connected to its delivery. His duties include implementation of policy decisions, informing the board of facts relating to policy questions, preparation of operating budgets, and maintenance of good community and personnel relations.

The Medical Staff—Historical

The key to the success or failure of hospital strategy is the staff physician. His position with regard to medical care is unique in the hospital and in society. Historically, doctors became involved with early hospitals as an act of charity in the community. The doctor's source of income was the paying private patient, who came to his office or was treated in the home. These conditions continued until changes in medical practice were brought about by scientific discoveries in anesthesia, asepsis, diagnostics, and the like. Such changes created the need for special equipment and trained assistants that were impossible for the physician to provide on an individual basis. Though the doctor has always been in charge of the care received by his patients—in or out of the hospital, paid or philanthropic—he has not been a force in the founding, development, or control of hospitals. This curious historical relationship is responsible for many of the difficulties in the trustee-administrator-doctor policy triangle. Since the physician-patient relationship is basic to an understanding of the doctor's role in the hospital, a pause is in order here to consider the unique legal entity known as the *practice of medicine.*

Society has long recognized that a person who dedicates his life to treating the sick deserves remuneration for his efforts regardless of his success or failure. There are conditions that cannot be improved no matter how skillful the physician. Some incentive should be provided the healer for his honest attempt to alleviate suffering; otherwise, he might be tempted to select for treatment only those cases having reasonable assurance of success, refusing to risk time and reputation where no guarantees could be given. Clearly, this would work to society's detriment. Borderline illness is the rule in medicine; and crisis intervention even under the best of conditions does not lend itself to certainty. Public interest is better served by encouraging the honest application of medical knowledge and skills and by requiring only the guarantee of conscientious effort.

The Medical Staff—Legal

Professional tradition, dating back to the third century B.C. and Hippocrates, ascribes to the doctor an unquestioned authority in matters pertaining to the care of his patient, subject only to the patient's consent. English common law and American case law have codified this tradition and have made explicit the doctor-patient relationship. The law defining the reciprocal agreement between healer and patient has taken on the character of business law: the practice of medicine is a personal service contract. As in all such contracts, four elements are essential to its validity: two contracting parties, a contractual object, a consideration, and mutual consent by the contracting parties. These are technical legal terms requiring definition by precedent case law and applicable statute. Obviously, precise definition is possible only for a given state, since both statutes and judicial decisions vary greatly from state to state. It is possible, however, to generalize for our purposes the usual understanding of these terms in relation to medical practice.

The parties involved are the doctor and the patient (or his legal guardian). Many situations occur wherein a physician is examining a person at the request of another party, such as an insurance company or a prospective employer. In such cases, the person has been held immune to suit for medical fees and doctors exempt from malpractice litigation, since no contract existed between the physician and the person treated. Any tangible, living human being with a real or imagined illness may be a patient, if one assumes he is legally competent. We thus exclude imaginary or dead persons and nonhuman creatures as parties to a contract for medical services.

The doctor involved must be a natural person with demonstrated qualifications in medicine and with the approval of the state to practice. A degree from a recognized school of medicine and a certificate of satisfactory completion of an accredited internship program are displayed in the physician's office as testimony to his knowledge and skill. Most states require a doctor to pass a written examination and have references from his instructors and peers in order to obtain a license to practice medicine. The natural person requirement means that a corporation cannot practice medicine. These, then, are the parties: a qualified physician with permission to practice and a human being with medical problems or complaints.

The object of medical practice is legal medical service with intent to benefit the patient. Performing illegal abortions, treating unreported gunshot wounds, resorting to euthanasia or sterilization, or using treatment methods prohibited by law do not constitute medical practice since the services rendered are illegal. Similarly, examination for the benefit of an insurance company, a trial court, or agency other than the patient examined does not qualify as medical practice.

Four activities are generally considered as uniquely medical activities: investigation, diagnosis, prescription, and therapy. Investigation is the determination of facts through laboratory tests, medical histories, measurements, and direct contact and observation. Diagnosis involves judging the nature of the disease on the basis of the skill and experience of the physician and also a review of all the facts produced by investigation. Prescription is the determination of the proper remedies for the disease. Therapy is the application of the prescribed remedies to the diseased person. Since investigation does not require the skill and judgment of a physician, many of the routine examination tasks may be carried out by trained assistants. Much of the usual therapeutic regimen is also of a routine nature and may be performed by anyone with the minimum of training, under qualified supervision. These activities are not part of the essential services involved in the practice of medicine. On the other hand, the diagnosis of a disease or condition and the prescription of a curative procedure are considered to require professional judgment beyond the knowledge of the ordinary citizen. They are the exclusive province of the qualified, licensed physician. They are the activities referred to as the object of medical practice.

Consideration in a personal contract is the motivation of each party to enter into the contract. This usually involves the delivery of a set of specified services for a fee that is agreed upon. In the case of medical services, the law does not require that any benefit accrue to the patient, nor need a physician provide any guarantee of the efficacy of the treatment prescribed. Usually, the law admonishes the physician against making any but the most general assurances, as do the canons of professional ethics of the American Medical Association. It is expected that the doctor will possess the necessary knowledge, skill, and judgment commonly associated with the physician and that he will apply himself to the best of his ability, holding as his primary goal the welfare of his patient. It is also expected that the medical services contracted for will be provided by the contracting physician. Any substitutes must be with the patient's permission.

In return for the conscientious application of the doctor's judgment, the patient is required by law to pay a reasonable fee. Many factors enter into a determination of what is reasonable. The training and professional experience of the doctor, the risks involved, the time required to treat the ailment, the difficulty of the treatment, the physician's standing in his profession, the seriousness of the disease or injury, and the accepted fee for that service by similarly qualified doctors in that location—all are factors to be considered. Under no circumstances is the outcome of treatment allowed to affect the fee. This is one of the staunchest canons of the medical profession.

Consideration is of prime importance in the medical practice contract. If there is no agreement as to the terms and amount of the consideration, the contract is void; however, the agreement need not be stated or written. Acceptance of services implies agreement to a reasonable charge for those services.

One of the most difficult areas of medical practice involves consent. Contract law requires mutual consent, by both parties freely given, to enter into a professional relationship before a contract can be considered valid. Consent may be implied or express. The doctor implies his consent to treat the public by hanging out his shingle; yet by the nature of the services offered, a doctor has the right to refuse to accept a patient. In practice, a refusal seldom occurs. The doctor with a full schedule or one who lacks some specialized skill will refer the patient to a colleague.

A patient also has the right to refuse medical care and to discharge or change his physician at his whim. His consent is implied as often as it is express. When a patient allows a doctor to examine and treat him without objection, his consent is implied. A written consent form is unnecessary.

The involvement of hospitals in much of the surgery performed today has created an interest on the part of hospital management that proper consent be obtained. For this reason, most hospitals require written consent forms to be signed by the patient before surgery is permitted in that hospital. The legal elements of consent are capacity or legal competence, understanding of the risks involved in the prospective treatment, and a free acceptance of those risks. Lack of competence because of age or mental condition will negate consent. Incomplete information or inadequate explanation of the risks involved will vitiate consent, and any fraudulent or coercive factors will cast doubt on its validity. If, for any reason, treatment is given to a patient without valid consent, the physician is subject to prosecution for battery or trespass upon the person so treated.

As the above statements suggest, the practice (or malpractice) of medicine is a concept requiring a great deal of judicial involvement. Medical law case books fill libraries, and medical schools provide courses and seminars on the legal status of medicine and the doctor vis-à-vis society. But the basic facts of medical practice are simple: given a live, human patient, of sound mind and common sense and complaining of pain or illness, the doctor may perform such legal treatment upon him as he deems valuable, with the patient's consent. The doctor is at all times in charge of the care of his patient, subject only to the terms of his contractual agreement with the patient.

The Medical Staff and the Hospital

We have been discussing the doctor's relationship to, and responsibility toward, the patient. What of his relationship to the hospital? What is his responsibility to the governing board or the medical staff of the institution? When the doctor's main source of income was the office patient, he was independent of hospital authority. As medical research has added "tools" to the doctor's bag (figuratively speaking), it has placed these tools more and more in the hands of hospital-paid and hospital-trained personnel. The doctor has become more and more dependent on hospital resources for the provision of specialized equipment, nursing care, and diagnostic procedures. Almost all serious surgery is performed in hospitals. The physician has had to relinquish some of his authority in order to cope with modern medical problems. At the same time, he has recognized the importance of the policy-making functions in determining his ability to care for his patients in the hospital environment in a manner he would consider optimum. Increasingly, doctors have become products of large medical school-teaching hospital complexes rather than of the apprentice methods of the past. All these factors enter into determining their role in the modern hospital.

The relationship of the practicing physician to his hospital has been described by Robert H. Guest, in his "Role of the Doctor," in six points:

1. The doctor is officially a guest of the institution, but his privileges are being limited by increasing pressures to conform to certain organizational constraints of the medical staff, the hospital, and third-party agreements.

2. The doctor is an independent professional, but he is becoming increasingly interdependent in his relations with his colleagues, other professionals, the administrator, and the governing authority of the institution.

3. The doctor makes his own financial arrangements with his clients, but these arrangements are to an increasing extent pre-established in schedules set up under health insurance and other third-party agreements.

4. The doctor has a fundamental right to minister to his client, the patient, but the responsibility for total patient treatment appears to be shifting toward greater involvement of other professionals, including the administrator.

5. The knowledge of clinical practice is "owned" by the doctor, but the technical tools of his practice are owned in large degree by the institution that gives him the privilege to practice. Even the doctor's clinical knowledge is being supplemented by specialized knowledge of other nonmedical members of the institution.

6. The doctor's role as a member of the hospital organization, as distinguished from his purely professional role, is being made increasingly explicit in bylaws of the medical staff and in written agreements with administrator, board, and outside parties of interest.[1]

Two additional factors tend to complicate the picture. First, many departments in the hospital are managed by doctors, who then become part of the administration, though not necessarily paid employees of the hospital. In any case, such a doctor becomes responsible for the organization and management of his department, the medical care of all patients treated under his supervision, and the enforcement of hospital rules. Many doctors are not prepared by training or inclination to be managers. The requirement to play a dual role continues to be a source of friction in many cases.

---

[1] From *Hospital Policy Decisions: Process and Action* (New York 1966) by Arthur B. Moss, Waune Broehl, Robert Guest, and John Hennessey, Jr., p. 181. By permission of G. P. Putnam's Sons.

Secondly, the doctor, in his professional life, belongs to several groups and associations external to, or beyond the control of, the hospital. These include the American Medical Association, the county medical association, and the medical staff organization of the hospital. It is in this latter group that the doctor makes himself felt most effectively in structuring institutional policy, though his position in extrahospital associations may color his views and bias his actions.

As a hospital guest, the physician accepts appointment to the hospital staff subject to all the rules and regulations thereto pertaining. His appointment grants him specific privileges of conducting certain medical procedures, depending on his skills, the hospital facilities, agreements with outside agencies, and the recommendations of the hospital staff. Credentials committees recognize that specialized procedures, such as neurosurgery, cardiac catheterization, and so forth, require training and skills beyond the competence of the ordinary MD. Thus, there is good reason for setting several levels of privilege and restricting staff members to those medical procedures in which they are competent. Many procedures, such as organ transplant and open heart surgery, are impossible without highly specialized equipment. The hospital lacking this equipment quite appropriately denies to its staff the privilege of performing the procedures.

The role of the doctor in his relation to the hospital is one of adaptation to an institution that has changed radically and continues to change under the pressure of a changing world. The physician has progressed far from the status of a voluntary, sometime visitor to an interdependent and influential member of the hospital organization. This has been often an unwilling mutation, and the institutional conflicts caused by the doctor's dual professional and administrative roles are not yet resolved. This is not intended as a criticism of the medical profession; on the contrary, the difficulties are such that one is amazed at the wealth of accomplishment of all facets of the hospital community. Such accomplishment is made possible by the continued dedication of all concerned to provide the best possible treatment for the sick and injured under their care.

The computer vendor must be sensitive to the dedication of all people connected with the community hospital. It is not possible to be successful either in selling or installing computer systems in the medical environment without an understanding of the basic motivations of the people involved. Business methods, cost displacement, efficiency, and the like are important to hospital administrators and boards of trustees; but even more important is their sense of service to the physicians and patients that utilize their institution.

BUDGET MAKING AS POLICY ACTION

It is instructive to examine relationships in another concrete example of policy formation, the creation of a hospital budget. In the previous chapter, the technical accounting aspects of the budget and financial control were discussed. Here we wish to examine mechanisms, procedures, and organizational relationships among the various interest groups involved in the budget process.

The budget process is understood to include the planning, coordination, and control of the income and expenses of all operating departments of the hospital. In this sense, hospital budgetary procedures are analogous to similar activities in industry. However, several factors—the lack of a profit motive, the inappropriateness of return-on-investment criteria, the unethical status of advertising and other attempts to increase the "share of the market"—make hospital budgeting a very different process in fact.

The institutional intent in budgeting is involved with the setting of priorities among the myriad goals; the allocation of chronically scarce resources; and the coordination of departmental, professional, and individual subgoals into a directed, coherent pattern. We have seen that the personal and professional ambitions of powerful individuals and groups in the hospital may not correspond exactly to institutional goals. The problem is aggravated by the failure of many hospitals to specify adequately what the primary institutional goals are and how each substratum of the hospital fits into the realization of these goals. Incomplete, conflicting, or overgeneralized goals are sources of much confusion and misunderstanding in achieving budgetary consensus.

In a larger sense, the hospital budget is more than a financial plan of operations. The budget should act as a gyroscope, maintaining equilibrium among the many conflicting forces and resolving those conflicts by economic pressure. Thus, the budget must be a dynamic instrument, modifying itself as the environment demands. It must be used as a mechanism for transforming goals into action. By assigning tasks and insisting on accountability, the hospital can form a set of dynamic coalitions to obtain specific benefits within and among departments. By using budgetary controls *on* expenditures to direct activities, the hospital can achieve the vital control *of* expenditures.

The budgetary process is initiated by the administration. A request is made of all department heads to prepare an estimate of the funds needed to operate their departments, including continuing activities, new services to be provided, pilot projects meriting investigation, and contingency emergency funds. The department heads are asked to estimate the income these activities will generate in their respective departments and also the sources of this income. The preparation of these preliminary budget figures becomes the subject of extensive interdepartmental discussion and may be brought up in several staff committee meetings as powerful interest groups compete for new equipment, additional personnel, or favored research project funding. At some specified deadline, the preliminary budget requests are returned to the administrator. It is his job to sell the budget to the board of governors, who must give final approval. He may find the budget requests unacceptable as presented. He may make modifications himself or return the preliminary budget requests to the department heads for corrections. In some hospitals both the board and the administrator prepare overall budgets separately, leaving departmental breakdowns for later discussions. These separate versions are then resolved by the board, which arrives finally at a budget acceptable to the administrator.

As the revision process continues, there is a matching and comparison of figures and a redefinition of goals. Conflicts in funding are resolved by discussions with the various department heads. As might be expected, the key personnel involved in budgetary policy decisions are the most influential members of staff, board, and administration. As economic constraints are evolved and communicated to the organization, issues affecting patient care are identified. The constraints and their effects on hospital goals are made explicit, and these are balanced against the opportunities for increased services and the risks of economic loss or loss of public support. The resulting budget is recognized by all to be an attempt at a consensus. The degree to which the budget meets the real needs of the hospital, coupled with the extent to which agreement has been reached among the special interest groups, determines the validity and usefulness of the budget.

Several studies regarding the budgeting process have been performed, all tending to reach the same basic conclusion: the professional status and hierarchical position of the influential members of the hospital with respect to budgetary matters the official relationships are rather clear cut because of the good budgets are produced as often as not by individuals of moderate professional standing and low hospital rank. The organization chart does not specify completely the power structure of the hospital. Still, position and status are factors to be considered. An understanding of the relationships of the various hospital factions, official and unofficial, is basic to a grasp of policy making. In budgetary matters the official relationships are rather clear-cut because of the regulations governing budget approval, but unauthorized groupings may be equally important in actually deriving funds for a given purpose.

As in all policy matters, the board has the final say in the budget. The trustees are considered the guardians of finance, but too often local and national trends in hospital progress tend to be ignored in favor of "economy of operation." Both the medical staff and the administrator feel the need to extend hospital services and improve the quality of patient care. The board, too, may have altruistic leanings, but tends to view them in terms of economic constraints.

These are not truly opposing views as much as different sides of the hospital management coin. The difference is fostered by the common failure of boards of governors to define institutional goals explicitly in economic terms. Trustees seem to be of the opinion that the staff lacks interest in the financial affairs of the hospital. This is not a totally groundless opinion in some cases. Hospital boards have a responsibility to show the medical staff that the constraints placed upon their idealism spring from a desire to fulfill total institutional goals in a practical manner rather than from arbitrary miserliness.

The job of the administrator in preparing the budget is perhaps one of the most trying encountered in hospital management. His skill in defining economic considerations often must fill in for the board's lack of clarity. His salesmanship must be superb to derive a consensus and resolve the numerous conflicts, and he must possess consummate skill as a manager to guide the hospital toward its goals while maintaining the desired budgetary controls. He sits squarely in the middle of the financial tug-of-war between the board and the medical staff. The ability to walk this tightrope is one of the characteristics of the good administrator.

Two attitudes characterize the members of the medical staff of the average community hospital. The first is jealousy of the attention given to their skill and judgment in matters medical. The second is a tendency toward exaggerated concern for patient care, expressed in a desire for expensive diagnostic or treatment facilities. Many physicians seem convinced that no one really cares about the patient but his doctor, and every physician believes that no one knows as well as he what is needed by his patients. That these attitudes color his relations with other members of the hospital policy team is obvious. They may also affect his ability to operate within the guidelines of even the wisest budget.

Much can be done to alleviate the problem by clear, explicit statements on financial policy by the board. If the members of the medical staff have the confidence of the board, it is likely they will have confidence in the board; but a realistic attitude on the part of the more insecure members of the staff is needed also. The essential sincerity and honest concern for patient care quality by all hospital officers must be recognized. Medicine has become too large and too specialized to be the private reserve of a few self-appointed guardians. The doctor is dependent on the skills and knowledge of many nonmedical professionals for assistance in diagnosis and therapy. Health care more than ever before requires teamwork. Fear of change and excessive regard for status are out of place in a profession devoted to care of the sick and injured.

As an example of the policy-making process, the preparation of the budget brings out the essential strengths and weaknesses of hospital organization and power structures. The diversity of backgrounds and interests of the members of the policy team insures a rich supply of ideas and creative methods of attack on the problems of hospital management. Yet the same diversity fosters conflicts and power struggles that threaten on occasion to rend the fabric of the health care system. That such men have been able to develop policies for administering the world's largest health care delivery system is a tribute to their dedication; that the system has failed to grow with the need for services created by an urban technological society is partially a reflection of the fragmented nature of the system itself and of the insecurities of some of its members.

Typical of the policy problems handled by the hospital are budgets. Budgets are a great problem in the hospital because funds are chronically scarce, often to such a degree that important health care programs must be curtailed.

Yet the members of boards of trustees and of the medical staff they govern are among society's most affluent people. In another sense, then, budgetary problems in the hospital reflect problems in the community and in society as a whole. As in most great social ventures, aspirations are larger than available resources.

SUMMARY

We have tried to describe the aims and mechanisms of hospital policy and also the persons responsible for its formation. We have attempted to answer several questions concerning hospital policy:

1. What are the concerns of policy in the hospital?
2. Who are the people influential in, and responsible for, hospital policy formation?
3. What are the mechanisms by which policy matters are determined?

The answers, as we have discovered, are not as definite as we might like. Hospitals are being forced to concern themselves with the social and economic problems of the outside world to a greater extent than ever before. External effects on hospital operations are growing at an ever-increasing rate, a fact that appears alarming to hospital management. The complex administrative structure of the voluntary hospital makes definitive policy procedures almost impossible to specify.

We have seen that one possible characterization of the policy-making process is that of dynamic resource allocation. We have said that all hospital resources, in the final analysis, are derived from society. In this view, a good hospital strategy is one that satisfies the real or imagined needs of the medical staff while remaining within the budget guidelines of the board. Clearly, many difficult questions are left unanswered in a short examination such as this.

Our example of data processing as a policy question left us with the same paradox. In fact, the question of computerization can point up the ambiguities and weaknesses of hospital policy mechanisms more quickly than the size of the expenditure would indicate. Few topics can elicit the emotional response in a hospital to compare with that caused by a suggestion to buy a computer. The reasons for this are not clear, but some hints can be found in the pervasiveness of computer activity in a medical setting and the professional jealousies of the people involved. It is well recognized that the computer will affect everyone in the hospital, though the nature and magnitude of the effects are not appreciated. The inclination of both the administration and the medical staff is to strive for control. However, more likely, the major reason is simply the basic conservatism of medicine, which quite rightly considers new technologies dangerous until clinical trials have proven them safe and effective. Computers in their short history of application to the hospital have not yet been exposed to sufficient "clinical" trials to satisfy the more cautious doctors and administrators.

We have not answered all of our questions concerning policy decisions and their effect on data processing, but we have uncovered some of the problems to be studied, and we have met the people involved in the decisions and learned something about how they interact. We shall find these data vital to an understanding of the environment in which our work as hospital information-processing specialists must be done.

REFERENCES

Eisele, C. Wesley. *The Medical Staff in the Modern Hospital.* New York: McGraw-Hill Book Co., 1967.

Guest, Robert H. "The Role of the Doctor." In *Hospital Policy Decisions: Process and Action.* New York: G. P. Putnam's Sons, 1966.

Letourneau, Charles U. *The Hospital Medical Staff.* Chicago: Starling Publications, 1964.

6

The Therapy System

INTRODUCTION

The previous chapters have treated the nonpatient-oriented hospital systems—service, building, supply (with a nod of exception for pharmacy), and management. From the point of view of patient care, these are support activities, important only to the degree that they improve or augment the treatment of ill and injured patients in the hospital. We have found that these support systems differ very slightly from their industrial counterparts. In this chapter we examine the main function of the hospital; its position as the focus of most of the health care in our society and also the activities carried out in satisfying patient care needs mark the distinguishing features of the hospital as an institution. This chapter is devoted to a discussion of the therapy system, which subsumes all those functions relating to the treatment of the ill and injured

There are many ways to view patient care activities in the hospital and the people dedicated to its services. Many valuable hours may be spent perusing some of the books listed at the end of this chapter. Here, we will follow our established pattern of observing the hospital from a systems viewpoint with special emphasis on the generation and use of information. Figure 6.1 describes the subsystem functional breakdown adopted in subsequent paragraphs.

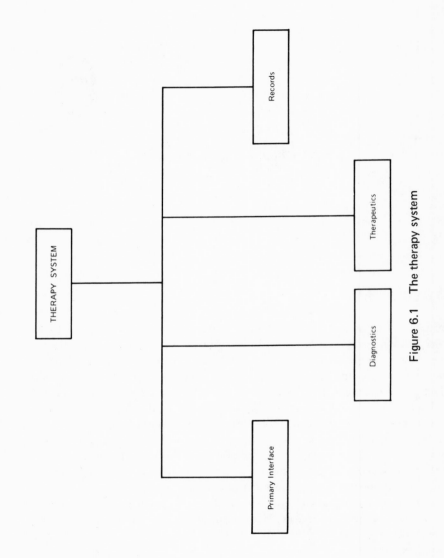

Figure 6.1 The therapy system

THE PRIMARY INTERFACE

If one considers the activities of other parts of the hospital as being supportive of the basic medical functions, then clearly there must be a mechanism by which the support functions are obtained and through which performance and charge data and other administrative information may be transmitted; that is, support functions must have an *interface* with medical functions. Much of this interface mechanism is of a purely communications-oriented nature and will be the subject of the next chapter; however, a few of these interface activities involve the actual movement of people and supplies and are included here under the title "Primary Interface." The consideration of these noninformation tasks is a departure from our usual methods. It is included here for completeness. There may seem to be some repetition of previous material, but the different orientation should become evident.

Primary interface activities take the patient from the outside world through the business management areas into the nursing wards and treatment areas and back out into the world again. They also are responsible for the movement of supplies from stores, central supply, and pharmacy up to the wards. We may call these activities *admissions and discharge* and *distribution*.

Admissions and Discharge

The importance of the admissions function to the proper care of the patient cannot be overestimated. The medical information gathered here can be extremely helpful if it is complete and accurate, but very misleading, possibly dangerously so, if not. The public relations value of a warm, cheery atmosphere and a helpful and understanding clerk at the admissions desk is immense. Good management also begins in admissions. Proper interviewing techniques secure the data needed to evaluate the legal and financial problems presented by every hospital patient. Mistakes made here, either of commission or omission, can be very costly to the hospital and unpleasant for the patient. The qualifications and training of admissions clerks should be given the same meticulous care that is used in the case of a lab technician or purchasing agent.

In chapter 2 we described some of the information-processing aspects of admissions. Here we will emphasize the movement of people through the system. There are three types of admissions commonly in use in the hospital. Each has its own procedures and protocols. The first is the emergency admission, which occurs because of an accident or natural disaster or because of the sudden onset of an illness, such as a coronary occlusion or an appendicitis attack. The important feature is the unplanned nature of the admission. In these cases, the patient most often arrives at the hospital emergency ward by ambulance. Here he is examined to discover the nature and severity of his problem. If no serious illness or injury requiring hospitalization is present, the patient is treated and sent home. If more extensive treatment or further study is required and if the patient meets the admissions criteria of the hospital, he is admitted to one of the wards. Admissions criteria are a matter of hospital policy and legal obligations. They may be economic, religious, or administrative; that is, age, sex, or special medical criteria may be set by some hospitals. There may be space problems in a particular hospital. In any event, if the patient is not acceptable to this hospital, he is moved to a more suitable one as soon as his condition permits safe transportation.

The second type of admission refers to an illness of sufficient severity to require immediate treatment, but not of emergency character. Such patients are usually referrals from staff physicians, who have discovered serious problems in the course of an office visit that require hospitalization for proper diagnosis and treatment. The same admissions criteria apply here as for emergency cases; however, since the admitting physician is on the hospital staff, the likelihood of an unacceptable patient is greatly reduced. According to the severity of the problem, the patient arrives in an ambulance or by private or public transportation.

The third type of admission is called preadmission and consists of patients whose conditions have a sufficiently long and predictable course that a time can be set for admission at the convenience of the doctor and patient. Such things as normal pregnancies, elective surgeries, periodic physical examinations, and the like, fall into this category. The planned nature of these admissions allows the hospital to prepare its records in advance, reserve space for the patient, and assure compliance with all admissions criteria. The better usage of resources encouraged by preadmissions makes this practice very desirable from the hospital management's viewpoint.

In all types of admission, the patient arrives at the hospital by some means of transportation and provides some minimum items of data for the admissions department. At this point, the movement of the patient is much the same for all. A nurse places the patient on a wheeled carrier, a stretcher, or a wheelchair, and rolls him to his assigned ward. There, he is undressed, his personal property is stored, and he is put to bed in his assigned location. A great deal of information transfer goes on attendant to the movement of the patient and the assignment of a room, but the primary interface has accomplished its mission once he is properly bedded down.

The discharge function is in many ways a mirror image of admissions. The movement of the patient is from his bed to the lobby and then out to the street, all by hospital wheelchair. There is a kind of debriefing, in which certain data are taken and certain instructions are given. Moreover, a great flow of communication takes place among the various departments related to the closing of accounts, the collection of last-minute lab results, and the availability of a bed for a new patient.

We shall return to the discharge and admissions functions in a later chapter, when we discuss information exchange and automation. We may conclude our discussion of patient flow through the admissions and discharge subsystem with a further reflection on patient movements within the hospital, unconnected with admission or discharge, but of necessity under the cognizance of that subsystem. Patients are moved around the hospital for many reasons: to go to a treatment area, to receive a diagnostic procedure, to have exercise or recreation, or to change bed or ward. All but the last are temporary; the patient will return to his bed shortly. Temporary movements are not important to the admissions and discharge subsystem. Permanent relocations occur for serious purposes, such as a change in the patient's condition requiring more or less intensive nursing care, or for frivolous ones, such as incompatibility with neighboring patients. Some moves occur because of a need for space in a particular area. In any event, since admission beds are assigned by the admissions and discharge subsystem, it is vital that the admit desk be aware of all changes in patient locations.

Distribution

We have discussed the distribution of supplies and prescriptions under the heading "The Supply System." We noted there that the two basic methods of distribution were the requisition method and the complement method. Our emphasis here is on the relationship between the physical delivery mechanisms, whether mechanical, electromechanical, or human, and the patterns of patient care in the hospital.

Nursing functions depend to a great degree on the availability of medical supplies in a timely fashion. The same can be said of surgery and many other areas of patient care. This is to state the obvious. It is perhaps not so obvious how much of the patient care profile in the wards is designed around the faulty, late, and inefficient supply services available from outmoded systems of distribution. Much of the waste of materials, overstocking of floor stocks, duplication of orders, and loss of charges occurs because the system of distribution is undependable. This causes a tendency to try to second-guess the system in order to insure service to the patients and avoid inconvenience to the staff.

It is possible to design a distribution system that does not suffer from these shortcomings. This does not imply excessive automation, extreme changes in patient care methods, or large expenditures. It does imply a commitment on the part of hospital personnel at all levels to make the system work; that is, to develop effective procedures and utilize them in their intended manner and to modify them where necessary to insure service. The savings in professional time and the improvement in patient care are worth the effort.

DIAGNOSTICS

We may now return to our customary procedures, analyzing information inputs, outputs, and internal processing. The reader may recall our functional description of diagnostics from chapter 2. Its purpose is to discover the nature and extent of the disease or injury. In an information-processing sense, symptomatic data and doctor's observations are input, tests are performed that generate new data, the totality of information is correlated and evaluated, and a diagnosis is output. The exact nature of the data generated depends upon the particular diagnostic procedures involved. For our purposes, we may classify the diagnostics subsystem into radiology, pathology, and special procedures. It should be noted that these classes may not correspond exactly to a hospital department of that name. A great deal of primarily diagnostic activity goes on in the separate treatment areas, and much of the internal processing of diagnostic data takes place in the mind of the physician. The complex and involved mental processes that make up this internal processing are quite beyond the scope of this book.

Radiology

The radiology subsystem is encompassed almost entirely in the radiology department. The functions of this department include treatments by therapeutic X ray and radioactive materials as well as the diagnostic usage of radiation. Radiology diagnostics always occur as a referral from the attending physician and produce results that must be interpreted by a radiologist and evaluated in the light of other diagnostic findings by the physician.

Three kinds of radiological diagnostic procedures are common. The first is the usual X-ray photograph, in which radiation is allowed to pass through some area of the body and be captured on film. The result is a shadow picture, the light and dark areas of which depend on the density of the tissues through which the rays must pass. Interpretation of X-ray films is a task requiring a great deal of skill and experience.

Fluoroscopy, the second type of diagnostic procedure, replaces the film with a radiation-sensitive screen and adds an opaque substance, either by mouth or intravenously, to the portion of the body being investigated, thus increasing the contrast of relevant features. One of the major benefits of the fluoroscope is the opportunity it provides to view deep structures in motion, isolate positions of diagnostic value, and record them on film by ordinary X-ray techniques.

The third kind of procedure may be called radioscanning. It involves the injection of one of a number of radioisotopes with very short half-lives. The substance chosen tends to gravitate to, or be absorbed by, a particular area of the body. For example, in the diagnosis of thyroid difficulties, a quantity of radioactive iodine is injected and subsequently absorbed by the thyroid gland; the percentage absorbed is a reliable measure of thyroid activity. A radiation counter is used to scan the area and derive a quantitative measure of radiation absorption.

The input to the radiology subsystem is in all cases a request form signed by a staff physician to perform a particular diagnostic procedure for a particular patient on a particular day. The request may involve detailed instructions concerning the physician's suspicions, specific anatomic features of interest, or items of medical history that may assist the radiologist in determining the most effective procedures to obtain the desired results. More often, the request contains no more than a simple statement of the series desired.

The output consists of several items of interest to the doctor and a brief statement of services performed for accounting purposes. The radiologist prepares a report, giving his expert opinion concerning the meaning of the data and results. This report, along with the films, radioscans, and other raw data, is made available to the requesting physician for his evaluation. In most cases, the physician will consult with the radiologist in person or by telephone concerning the interpretation of his findings.

Internal processing depends to a degree on the kind of procedure requested. Some of the steps, such as those related to processing the request, scheduling the procedure, and the like, are common throughout the department. Others relate to the interpretation of results and their communication to the physician. Let us follow these steps in sequence from the moment a request enters the department.

First, the patient must be scheduled, preferably on the day requested by the physician. This is not always a simple process. Many factors external to the department have large effects on its activity. For example, many radiological procedures are invalidated by diet, drugs, or injections used in other diagnostic procedures. This means that a knowledge of the patient's total activity for at least a 24-hour period prior to his appointment in X ray is necessary to insure proper test results.

In addition, scheduling problems may occur in the system itself. There may be no available time on the day requested by the doctor either because of heavy activity in the X-ray department that day or because personnel or equipment are not functioning. This necessitates a conversation with the doctor and perhaps a rescheduling of several days' activity for his patient. The sequence in which tests are scheduled may be very important. A chest X ray followed by a skull series, followed by another chest film, may require 25 percent more time than the same procedures with the two chest X rays grouped together because of the machine setup time. Increased productivity in the X-ray department reduces both patient waiting time and departmental costs.

If these difficulties can be surmounted and the patient can be scheduled, a notice is sent to his ward giving detailed instructions concerning his activity on the day preceding his test. There are directions telling him how to get to the X-ray area if he is ambulatory. On the day of his appointment, the well-run radiology department will check with the ward to be sure everything is in order and to remind ward personnel that the patient is expected. This can reduce the number of missed appointments and wasted resources.

When the patient arrives, his identification is checked, along with the test scheduled and any factors that might affect the procedure adversely. After an appropriate waiting period in which the patient may contemplate the wonders of modern medicine, the patient is disrobed and taken to the test area. There the indicated procedures are performed, data are collected, and a record is made of the gross facts and appearances of his test. At this point, the patient is asked to wait until the technician is sure that a valid test result has been obtained.

The data collected in their raw form have little meaning for the average physician. The radiologist is a doctor who has specialized in the interpretation of radiological procedures. His function is to review the test data for the requesting physician, to point out salient features and their meaning, and to suggest possible diagnoses based on the test results for the attending physician's consideration. The radiologist writes a report summarizing his findings and holds a personal conference with the physician in important cases. This report constitutes the major output of the radiology subsystem.

After the test is performed and valid results obtained, clerical personnel fill out a charge slip detailing the procedure performed, the date and time, and the patient's indentification number, for use by the business office. This slip, along with utilization statistics and departmental activity reports, makes up the remainder of the output from this subsystem.

A few hospital departments have X-ray and radioscanning equipment that is used independently of the radiology department. Examples are urology, neurology, and dentistry. This is usually specially designed equipment of little value outside its intended use. The information-processing activities are not greatly affected by the location of the equipment except that the requesting physician acts as his own radiologist.

Pathology

There are many diseases that may be diagnosed and treated at earlier stages by laboratory tests, thus improving the prognosis. Some diseases scarcely could be diagnosed at all without the services of the laboratory. In addition, the course of treatment of a disease may be monitored and results verified by clinical laboratory examinations. All these things make the pathology subsystem one of the most valuable in the hospital.

There are two basic divisions in pathology. The first, anatomical pathology, is the study of the structural and functional changes in the tissues and organs of the body that cause or are caused by disease. This is often an experimental or research activity, though, as in all medical research, it may lead to useful information for the practicing physician. The second division, clinical pathology, forms the major topic of this section. It deals with the actual observation and treatment of patients. Clinical pathology is the study of the various laboratory procedures, tests, examinations, tissue cultures, and other analyses pursuant to the diagnosis and treatment of real patients in live situations. The typical pathology laboratory has six units: hematology, serology, biochemistry, bacteriology, urinalysis, and histology.

Hematology Unit. Hematology is the study of the structure and gross anatomy of the blood and blood-forming tissues. The kinds of tests performed include counting of blood cells and other particulate matter in the blood; coagulation and sedimentation rates; and hematocrit, the percentage of red cells in whole blood. These tests are useful in diagnosing numerous disease conditions, including all types of infections, liver damage, and clotting mechanism abnormalities.

Serology Unit. This unit is named for its preoccupation with antigen-antibody reactions that take place in serum, the clear liquid left when blood coagulates. Certain foreign proteins, called antigens, stimulate the formation of chemically related substances, or antibodies, when introduced into the serum. Antibodies are an important part of the body's defense mechanism against disease. The tests performed in this unit include antigen analysis, antibody classification, albumin-globulin ratio, and blood typing. These tests and many others performed in the serology unit assist in the diagnosis and treatment of allergies, irregularities in antibody formation, and Rh factor complications, as well as being of immeasurable value to the blood bank.

Biochemistry Unit. Biochemistry is the chemistry of physiological processes. Many diseases foster changes in the fluids and tissues of the body that can be best detected by biochemical analysis. The tests performed include hydrolysis, colorimetry, photometry, gas chromotography, and reagent-reaction tests. From these tests the doctor can discover how well the body metabolizes sugar, how much oxygen the lungs can extract from the air, what percentage of usable protein is in the blood, as well as many other facts relating to the overall functioning of physiological processes.

Bacteriology Unit. This unit is concerned with the effects on the body of bacteria and their toxins. All tests in this unit start with a culture, which is a growth of bacteria in a specially prepared culture medium. A sample containing bacteria is placed in the medium and allowed to grow until colonies of sufficient size are present to perform the requested procedures. The samples may come from blood, urine, stools, sputum, or other fluids or tissues. There are several kinds of tests performed on the bacteria cultures: agglutination, antibiotic sensitivity, fluorescent antibody tests, special tests for parasitic infections, and so forth.

Urinalysis Unit. Most of the tests performed on the urine have to do with the functions of the urinary tract, kidneys, bladder, and so forth. However, some tests in this unit measure conditions in other organs or are used to detect other systemic diseases by their effect on the contents or character of the urine. These diseases include diabetes, severe heart failure, drug toxicity, bone tumors, liver malfunction, electrolyte imbalance, and lead poisoning. Urine tests also form the most reliable early tests for pregnancy.

Histology Unit. Histology is the study of the microscopic structure and composition of the tissues. Surgical and autopsy specimens are viewed, and slides are prepared that may be examined by microscope by a pathologist. This is the only unit that requires the services of the pathologist. Of course, he should direct the efforts and review the results of all units, but only in histology must he be personally involved. The tests performed consist of nothing more dramatic than staring through the microscope's eyepiece. Yet most malignant tumors are diagnosed here, and no postmortem is complete without a histologic work-up.

In many hospitals the blood bank is part of the pathology laboratory since blood typing requires many of the standard laboratory procedures. In this case, facilities are needed for transfusions, for the drawing of blood from donors, and for the proper storage of blood. The average hospital cannot supply all its needs for whole blood and plasma. Usually, the hospital contracts with one of the nonprofit corporations that supply blood in quantity.

The input for the pathology subsystem is analogous to that of the radiology subsystem, consisting of physicians' requests for a particular set of tests. The major difference between them lies in the volume of requests received and tests per week performed. In a 300-bed hospital, 9,000 tests will be performed in the laboratory, as compared with about 3,000 X rays.

Pathology output is also similar to its radiology counterpart, but laboratory data are generally more easily quantified. Test results are often in the form of percentages, cell counts, grams or cubic centimeters, or readings from a scale. Thus, they lend themselves to more traditional data-processing methods. We shall see in subsequent chapters how much difference this makes in attempts to automate functions within these two subsystems. Histology output data are the exception in pathology; they have much the same form as in radiology—a report in medical terminology of the pathologist's findings.

Internal processing, as far as information is concerned, also follows similar steps in this subsystem. One fact, however, stands out in the movement of patients; a large percentage of patients do not come to the laboratory for the tests or to draw samples. The complications arising because of this fact more than outweigh the simplifications. Since patients are staying in their wards, there are not the scheduling and waiting problems encountered in radiology. On the other hand, samples must be obtained from patients who may move around or be improperly identified. The following paragraphs describe the changes that must be made in the internal processing steps.

The physician's request arrives in the ward as before. The requests are sorted by ward and room, and a sample "drawing list" is made up that details the kind and amount of each sample needed. A technician is dispatched at regular intervals to pick up the samples. Occasionally, the ward personnel will have drawn the sample. If not, the technician checks his list and draws the amount of liquid required. The samples are returned to the laboratory, matched with the requests, and divided into a sufficient number of portions for the tests requested. Then they are sorted by unit and work station. As the tests are completed, the data are collected on test result sheets, charge slips are prepared, and a report is made up for the requesting doctor.

The above procedures assume that all tests are requested in plenty of time for the drawing, sorting, collecting, and testing operations to be completed and for the results to be made available to the physician. Often this is not the case. Patient conditions change rapidly with some diseases; accidents and emergency onsets of illness, such as appendicitis and heart attacks, require immediate treatment. In such situations, test results are needed as soon as possible. These tests are sent to the lab with the sample and marked STAT (abbreviation of the Latin *statim* "immediately"). In other cases, clerical workloads and inefficient data handling may result in the late arrival or processing of requests. This means an extra routing of technicians to draw samples if the test reports are to be ready on time. More often, rerouting is not possible, and the tests must wait until the next day. Impatient physicians, faced with poorly designed information procedures, are tempted to mark all their tests STAT, thus further complicating the situation. The number of tests not channeled through the regular procedures can reach significant proportions, fully half of all tests in some hospitals.

Special Procedures

There are several diagnostic tests that do not fit into the two previous classes. They are designed for special medical problems. Very few patients are given these tests. Generally, the attending physician in cases requiring these "special procedures" are themselves specialists and are qualified to administer and interpret them. There are few formal inputs or outputs. The doctor decides when and if a patient requires a given test and proceeds to schedule and administer it. The data derived from the test are interpreted immediately, often as the test is being given; and the implications are integrated into the patient's therapy. The only record of the test may be the doctor's informal notes.

As in other diagnostic tests, the internal processing depends primarily upon the type of procedure involved. The tests in this special category include electroencephalography, electrocardiography, electromyography, phonocardiography, cardiac ballistics, angiography, and cardiac catheterization. As the names indicate, most of the special procedures are based on electrophysiological or radiological techniques. The technology used is new, and the degree of automation for recording, controlling, and interpreting the tests is high. This is a fertile

PATIENT NAME

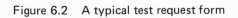

" X " BOXES WITH BALL-POINT PEN
TO INDICATE REQUEST. PRESS DOWN

☐ STAT	☐ ROUTINE	☐ 24 HRS	COMP DATE	/ /
DATE OF REQUEST		REQUESTED BY:	TECHNOLOGIST	

INFORMATION

☒	← C B REQUEST	TEST		RESULTS	
		SOURCE			
☐		AFB CULTURE			
☐		BLOOD CULTURE			
☐		MISC CULTURE			
☐		SMEAR			
☐		P & O (WET MOUNT)			
☐		OCCULT BLOOD			
☐		SENSITIVITY R=RESISTANT S=SENSITIVITY		R	S
		- CHLORAMPHENICOL			
		- FURADANTIN			
		- GANTRISIN			
		- KANAMYCIN			
		- MANDELAMINE			
		- GARRAMYCIN			
		- NALIDIXIC			
		- POLYMIXIN B			
		- CHOLYMYCIN			
		± OLEANDOMYCIN			
		± AMPICILLIN			
		± CEPHALOTIN			
		± DIHYDROSTREPTOMYCIN			
		± ERYTHROMYCIN			
		± TETRACYCLINE			
		+ LINCOMYCIN			
		+ METHICILLIN			
		+ PENICILLIN			
		+ OXACILLIN			
		+ CLOXACILLIN			

BACTERIOLOGY
CHART

Figure 6.2   A typical test request form

area for computer applications. In the next chapters we will discuss some of these applications.

THERAPEUTICS

The medical areas included in therapeutics are indeed the most important in the therapy system in the entire hospital. There are many ways to classify the functions and activities included under the title *therapeutics*. We may look at the departmental organizations. We may examine the medical specialties. For our purposes, however, information processing still provides the most fruitful division. In observing the kind of data generated, the information needed for proper functioning, and the way in which data are used, an almost automatic division occurs: medicine, surgery, and nursing. It is well here to remind the reader again that our classifications do not correspond in all particulars to the hospital departments or medical specialties of the same name. They are abstractions the value of which depends on their ability to clarify the information-handling tasks in the hospital. We shall define what we mean by each of them in the following paragraphs and how they are related to the various medical activities of the hospital.

Medicine

The medicine subsystem consist of all those functions usually performed by the physician, excluding surgical procedures. Remembering the definition of medical practice from a previous chapter, we may quickly derive the characteristics of this subsystem. It includes those activities known as diagnosis, or the determination of the agency causing the patient's symptoms, and prescription, or the selection of a curative regimen for the disease condition. A word is in order concerning the difference between the diagnostic functions of this subsystem and the functions of the diagnostics subsystem of the previous sections. The diagnostics subsystem provides the data and their medical meaning from its many tests and diagnostic procedures. The medicine subsystem transforms data, interpretations, consultative reports, and suggestions into a diagnosis.

There are many medical specialities the functions of which are part of this subsystem. A partial list includes internal medicine, psychiatry, neurology, cardiology, dermatology, obstetrics, pediatrics, urology, epidemiology, gynecology, orthopedics, geriatrics, and tropical medicine. To describe these fields with any completeness would require a library of medical textbooks. However, there are many similarities in the information-handling aspects of these specialties. Let us examine the internal processing, input, and output as the doctor practices his profession.

The input to the medicine subsystem consists of all the known facts concerning the patient and his condition. These facts come from a medical history, test results from the diagnostics subsystem, physical examination and observation, and comments from consulting specialists. The sequence of input and the kind of test performed are determined by the physician as he relates each fact to what he knows of the patient and the possible disease conditions he may have. Often, the physician is able to diagnose a problem with no more than a thorough physical examination. In rare cases, the full battery of tests available through the diagnosis subsystem is required.

The main output desired is a diagnosis, an explanation of the objective test results and doctor's observations, and a statement of the cause of the symptoms. The human body is a physiological system of incredible complexity and a high degree of intersystem relationship. The malfunction of any one part affects the workings of every other part; therefore, a diagnosis can seldom be perfect in the sense that it explains all the known facts. The doctor must be satisfied with a partial or tentative diagnosis, which can be improved or verified as treatment continues.

The processing involved in converting the input data into an output diagnosis has many facets. In one sense, it is a form of multivariate pattern recognition. Tens or even hundreds of measurements and observations are correlated; and a pattern is evolved, a concise picture of the patient's condition, which may be compared with other patterns, patterns characteristic of particular diseases or injuries. In another sense, diagnosis requires a degree of intuitive judgment defying any systematic description, or so we are told. Much of the process by which a diagnosis is reached may be reduced to logical or mathematical procedures applied to measurable parameters characteristic of certain disease conditions; and much of it seems to be intuitive, creative, beyond rationality. It is necessary, on occasion, to guess or assume a diagnosis and treat the patient in terms of it, even in the absence of definitive test results. Some physicians believe that this is the norm in medicine rather than the exception. The hackneyed statement that medicine is an art is a recognition of this view.

The output of the diagnostic process forms the input for the prescription process. Often, there are several possible, mutually exclusive diagnoses. In many cases, there are several simultaneous and contributing illnesses or injuries. The input procedures must be able to distinguish all the possible combinations of tentative and simultaneous diagnoses.

The desired output of the prescription process is a set of curative or therapeutic measures designed to comfort, alleviate, or perhaps cure the input diagnoses. Because of the multiplicity of these diagnoses, the prescribed regimen may be quite complicated. The range of therapeutic methods available to the physician is extremely broad. It includes drugs, surgery, radiation, cryogenics, diet, rest or exercises, and any combination of these measures.

Again, the internal processing involved consists of equal parts of art and science, with a dash of pure witchcraft. Much of the therapy prescribed, even in modern medicine, appears to be the result of trial and error rather than definitive knowledge. This is partly due to the infinite complexity of human illness. In addition, not enough is known concerning such basics as cellular biochemistry, the effects of radiation and drugs, and the etiology of many diseases, such as arthritis. In the absence of this knowledge, the doctor has no choice but to follow his experience and judgment, that is, to guess. Even in those cases in which our understanding is fairly complete, there is a surprising inconsistency, a significant variability in response, to a given therapeutic measure among ostensibly similar patients. Under these conditions, any real certainty in prescribing for a particular patient with particular symptoms is impossible. The best that can be hoped for is that the prescription will be statistically justified. Faced with this situation, the physician is to be forgiven if he acts unscientifically, if he resorts to intuition, and if his treatment of patients is less than perfect.

The overall sequence of events in the diagnosis and prescription process may be summarized as follows:

1. A patient consults a doctor because of a problem he recognizes himself or at the suggestion of another physician.

2. The doctor begins the phase of data collection with a family history, a medical questionnaire, and a gross physical examination.

3. On the basis of what these may indicate and what the patient can tell him about the symptoms and sensations of his condition, the doctor forms a set of tentative diagnoses.

4. From the great number of tests and procedures available, the doctor selects those that he hopes will assist him in his diagnosis. Because of the cost, time, and inconvenience to the patient, the doctor should be careful to select only the number and type of tests needed for his diagnosis.

5. Armed with as many facts and observations as possible about the patient, the physician applies his experience, knowledge, and judgment to arrive at, or sometimes to guess at, a working diagnosis. This must be considered tentative until further observations and the results of therapy can verify the conclusions.

6. The physician then searches his mind, notes, and relevant medical literature for the proper course of treatment. Often, there are complications that may encourage him to seek consultation with his colleagues.

7. During the application of the chosen therapy, the patient's condition must be carefully monitored. Changes might be indicative of improvement, a bad reaction to therapy, or a necessity for further diagnostics.

The actual application of the chosen therapeutic measures is performed more often than not by nursing or technical personnel. We shall examine in a subsequent chapter some of the attempts at the automation of the diagnostic and prescription processes.

Surgery

Surgery is possibly the most dramatic aspect of medicine to the layman. Its history is almost as old as writing. Four thousand years ago in Egypt, rather complicated surgical procedures were performed, although under primitive conditions of anesthesia and asepsis. New developments in these areas have made possible some remarkable surgical procedures as well as the virtual elimination of the high mortality rates previously connected with surgery. Surgery has become one of the most glamorous of professions.

The importance of surgery in modern medicine can be seen from the fact that fully half of all hospital admissions result in some kind of surgery. The most frequently performed surgeries are episiotomies, circumcisions, tonsillectomies, adenoidectomies, appendectomies, and inguinal herniorrhaphies, in that order. As we define it in this chapter, surgery is a therapeutic measure rather than a diagnostic procedure. The department of surgery as a hospital staff organization functions in all areas of medicine.

One special area connected with surgery deserves mention. Anesthesiology has become so important and its procedures so complex that it has to be considered a medical specialty in its own right. Decisions concerning the use of the potent drugs required to induce and maintain anesthesia during surgery must be made by a qualified professional. In addition to his importance in matters medical, the anesthesiologist plays a vital role in the information-processing functions of the surgery subsystem.

The surgery subsystem enters the treatment picture usually after some relative certainty has been reached concerning a diagnosis. Surgery is one of many possible courses of treatment. Its unique importance to us derives from its frequency compared to other therapeutic measures carried out in the hospital and from the variety and complexity of its information-handling tasks.

Owing to the nature of surgical procedures, the input to the surgery subsystem is rather broad and varied. It includes all medical data collected by the other parts of the therapy system, diagnostic conclusions, consultative commentaries, and the entire gamut of physiological measurements and observations made during the actual operation.

The output is as limited as the input is varied. Most of the input to the surgery subsystem stops there; it is a data sink. Some of the medical information may be passed on in the form of entries to the medical record, and, of course, there is a results-of-surgery report. But for the most part, surgery makes internal use of the data, both input and generated, and provides very little information output.

The internal processing in the surgery subsystem is as complex as anywhere in the hospital. Data of all varieties come into the system, consisting of medical information concerning the patient, requests for facilities and personnel, and direct measurements during the operation. These data must be sifted and acted upon. Only by breaking down the incoming flood to a number of logical data streams can some sense be made of the overall processing. We may call these paths administrative, consultative, and physiological. Let us examine these data streams separately in a quasi-chronological sequence to determine their functions and interactions.

The administrative data stream consists of requests for surgical services, that is, requests to schedule a patient for a particular procedure on a certain day. This, in turn, requires specific facilities, personnel, and supplies, some of which must fulfill other surgical commitments on that day. The first processing task is to work all the procedures into the crowded schedule of available surgical suites and overworked OR nurses, anesthetists, and technicians. After the operation, a report must be made to the business office describing the supplies and facilities actually used in order to allow proper charging for services. In addition, the nursing staff or ward personnel must be alerted for the arrival of the postre-covery patient. Finally, the report of the surgical results and any other relevant data are added to the medical record.

The consultative data stream refers to the set of diagnoses, X rays, medical history, and comments by consulting physicians that assist the surgical staff in planning the surgery. This information is referred to throughout the procedure both as a guide and for corroborative evidence. If during the course of the operation unsuspected conditions are found that require further diagnosis and treatment, this information is fed into the data stream and continues through the surgery subsystem and back to the patient's physician, that is, to the medicine subsystem.

The physiological data path consists of all electrophysiological and me-chanical signals from the patient, such as EEG, EKG, pulse, blood pressure, and so forth, as well as observations of the patient by all OR personnel. Based on these data, various actions may be taken to assure the patient's anesthesia or to intercept potentially dangerous changes in his condition.

All these paths actually intertwine in the care of the surgical patient. Part of the information needed for proper scheduling is the medical data required to plan and perform the surgery. Observations during the procedure become part of the medical record and may also trigger further consultation. The physiological monitoring needed during surgery often continues throughout recovery and forms the basis for later nursing care. The surgeon, as the professional responsi-ble for all surgical activities, must correlate the data streams, guide the other surgical personnel, perform the actual operation, and make decisions concerning all aspects of the surgery subsystem.

Nursing

Of all hospital departments, the Department of Nursing has the most complex organization. Nursing has responsibility for the continuous care of the hospital's patients. There are very few areas or functions in the hospital that do not relate to nursing activities. Each of the medical departments has its own nursing staff reporting to the director of nursing. Operating room, emergency, maternity, nursery, and rehabilitation all have specially trained nursing personnel who also report to the director of nursing. The nursing staff constitutes the largest group of hospital employees, averaging more than one-half of the total hospital personnel complement. Nurses comprise more than 70 percent of all persons employed in health-related fields nationally. There are almost two million nurses and nurse's aides practicing in the United States, compared with 350,000 physicians.

Nursing personnel can be classified in three broad categories—registered or graduate nurses (RNs), practical or vocational nurses (LVNs), and nurse's aides and orderlies. Registered nurses are graduates of an approved educational and on-the-job training program and are required to pass a licensing examination conducted by the State Board of Nursing. They are responsible for the nature and quality of the care given to hospital patients and for carrying out physicians' instructions. They also supervise the activities of LVNs and other nonprofessional personnel performing routine ward duties. Educational programs leading to nursing diplomas are usually three or four years in length; but special fields such as operating room techniques, intensive and cardiac monitoring, or emergency procedures may take as long as six years.

Practical nursing licensure has been required in all 50 states since 1960. Again, an approved educational program and a state examination are mandatory. Training usually lasts about 18 months. LVNs provide nursing care and treatment of patients under the supervision of a registered nurse. Much of the routine treatment may be carried out by LVNs depending on the rules of the hospital. In some hospitals, LVNs may perform such techniques as drainage, irrigation, catheterization, and even medication. They are often responsible for taking and recording temperature, blood pressure, pulse, respiration, and liquid intake/ output.

Nurse's aides (usually women) and orderlies or attendants (usually men) function as assistants to the RN and LVN in providing for patient welfare and comfort. They perform the less skilled tasks of patient care, provide supportive and sanitary services, and handle the heavier nursing duties. They are required by law and good hospital procedures to be under close supervision by a registered or practical nurse at all times. Few hospitals have any definite educational requirements for nurse's aides, though on-the-job training and orientation programs are common.

For our purposes, the differences between the categories of nursing are not as important as the similarities. The nursing staff collectively generates by far the largest volume and variety of information in the hospital. The basic source of all information in the hospital is the patient, and the nurse is the primary hospital contact with that source. Data input and output in the nursing wards are enormously high in both amount and complexity. Before we proceed to examine the input/output and internal processing of the nursing subsystem, let us examine the information-processing tasks connected with the arrival, stay, and departure of a patient at a nursing ward.

1. The patient arrives at the ward at his prescheduled time. Admission forms have been filled out and sent to the ward, so that the admissions data input has been accomplished.

2. Surgical permission forms and various insurance forms are filled out, signed by the patient, and witnessed by ward personnel.

3. The ID bracelet or floor ID cards prepared by the admit desk are used to imprint orders, charts, and so forth. These are either waiting at the nursing station or brought up with the patient. The ward is often notified by telephone before the patient arrives.

4. The ID card is placed in a convenient rack according to bed location, and the patient's name is entered in the appropriate doctor's log. Several checks are made with the housekeeping, dietary, and laboratory departments to assure that the patient's name appears on their census lists.

5. Using the ID card, a clerk imprints the patient's name on a long list of documents, forms, charts, and records. A partial list follows: intercom directory, release from responsibility for belongings, nurse aide card, nurse card, Medicare certification, allergy record, physical examination form, laboratory reports form, nurse's notes form, progress notes form, and a variety of charge slips for all services delivered.

6. The doctor's orders are transcribed onto the appropriate form for his signature. Copies are made on the nurse's card, medication card, laboratory card, and charge slips. Then the entire bundle is placed in order on a clip board, one per patient. These become the beginnings of the medical record.

7. Thereafter, every action taken in reference to the patient and every observation made on the patient is recorded on the prepared forms. Hospital activities are very much time-oriented; that is, certain activities must occur at the same time every day. They are also extremely formalized, thus allowing for easy recording on the designed forms. The recording and transcribing tasks are one of the primary responsibilities of the nursing staff.

8. When the doctor ascertains that the patient is ready to go home, he informs the nursing ward. Ward personnel enter the patient's name on the daily transfer and discharge work sheet. When the patient is dressed and ready to leave, a discharge order is prepared and copies sent to admissions and the various other hospital departments.

Most of the above information-handling tasks are performed at the nursing station, the ward's information and communications center. There are many devices, visual, mechanical, and electronic, that assist the ward personnel in their data-processing and transmission duties. Telephones, bulletin boards, reference books, intercoms, alarm buzzers and lights, plastic card imprinters, charts, cardex files, voice recorders, and handout brochures are a few of these.

To summarize, the input to the nursing subsystem consists of admissions data, patient history and medical examination data, orders from staff physicians, and requests for services from the patients themselves. The output has many forms, from orders for patient services, to medical measurements and nursing notes, to charge data and discharge notices—everything that has to do with the care and progress of the patient in his stay on the ward. Internal processing in the nursing subsystem is mainly a matter of measurement and recording. Very little decision making by ward personnel is encouraged or allowed. Nursing provides the data; medicine and management make the decisions.

The above description is typical of the manual data-handling methods prevalent in today's hospitals. They have many drawbacks. Under this system, fully 60 percent of the working time of ward personnel is spent on paperwork. There are few hospitals with adequate feedback of scheduling and supply conflicts in their procedures for ordering treatments, lab tests, X rays, and the like. This causes excessive queuing and dangerously long waiting times. And most important, there is very little effective error control, either of patient care information or of charge data. Often no audit trails are provided. An error in identification can cause lost or mistaken medications and wrong interpretations of test results. In a sensitive area like the nursing ward, where most of the medical and accounting data are generated, there should be absolutely foolproof methods of data capture, recording, and communication. Manual methods have never been successful or cost effective in achieving these goals.

RECORDS

The records subsystem is classified here as part of the therapy system, since its main function relates to the improvement of patient care; however, the records subsystem is affected by, and has an effect on, every department, function, and activity in the hospital. Medical records are of major importance in the evaluation of performance of personnel and services. They are vital to attaining accreditation from the Joint Commission. They serve as a resource for educational programs at all levels. They are the basis and the verification of most of the research carried out in hospitals, and they form the body of knowledge of patient facts and observations without which treatment of patients would be impossible.

The medical record is a permanent documentation of the history and progress of a patient's illness or injury. It is meant to be a complete and comprehensive compilation of observations, measurements, notes, and findings from the time the patient is admitted until the time he is discharged. It is axiomatic that in order to fulfill these requirements, there must be a total dedication by the records subsystem to completeness and accuracy. Equally important, the records must be filed properly and easily accessible to authorized persons. Many people are responsible for the myriad forms, slips, and documents that are entered into the medical record. Admissions, the medical staff, nursing personnel—all have input to the system; but the basic responsibility belongs to the personnel, procedures, filing methods, and the records themselves that make up the records subsystem.

To be complete, the medical record must contain as a minimum the following data:

1. An abstract of the patient's family background, medical history, employment record, immunizations, and any other significant historical data

2. A detailed record of all physical examinations performed during the current incident of illness

3. All physical and physiological measurements, especially those made by persons other than the physician (These include height, weight, dimensions of body parts, pulse rate, temperature, respiration, arterial and venous blood pressure, EEG, EMG, EKG, blood gases, intraocular pressure, tongue fibrillation, reflexes, and many others.)

4. Measurements and test results of the patient's personality, emotional state, and intelligence

5. Measurements and test results taken from the various specimens of blood, urine, feces, sputum, and body tissues (These are usually the results of clinical laboratory procedures.)

6. A complete history of the course of the current incident, including original complaint, working diagnoses, tests performed, an explanation of the logic by which the diagnoses were reached, the treatment prescribed, the results of treatment, the current status and condition of the patient, and the probable prognosis.

It is tempting to view such an agglomeration of facts and opinions as comprehensive in the sense that all significant information concerning the patient and his problem is contained therein. In fact, that is not the case. A great deal of vital information is communicated among the various members of the health care team in conversations, informal notes, unspoken attitudes and gestures, and so forth. Most of this data is not and can never be recorded. Thus the record is doomed to some degree of information loss. The immense number of forms, requisitions, and authorizations, resulting in an inordinate amount of professional time spent on paper handling, is, in part, an attempt to capture as much as possible of the available data before they are lost or forgotten.

The input to the records subsystem can be considered the entire written output of the hospital, excluding most of the detailed accounting records. Copies of all the forms discussed in the primary interface, diagnostics, and therapeutics subsystems find their way here, as well as much of the information collected or generated by all the other hospital systems.

The output has varied forms, but in the main consists of patient-related or patient care-oriented information. It may be the complete record of a given patient, a portion of the record, or a composite of many cases of interest to hospital management. It may relate to patient care improvements, the research project of a member of the medical staff, a review of hospital personnel and procedures, or the hospital's educational program. The format, content, and quantity of data will depend upon the use intended for the information.

There are a variety of internal processing tasks carried out by the records subsystem. Often these tasks are vital to the completeness and usefulness of the records. One of them refers directly to completeness. Records personnel spend a great deal of time cajoling the medical staff into keeping the records of their patients current. Occasionally, it becomes necessary to bring the status of incomplete records to the attention of hospital management. Possibly no other single violation of accreditation standards is as frequent as incomplete or otherwise unsatisfactory medical records.

Most of the internal processing in the records subsystem is designed to make references and retrievals of the information more reliable, easier, and quicker. Diseases and injuries by type are the most common key for reference by researchers and medical staff members. Here the problem lies in the ambiguity or duplication of terminology. There is sufficient argument among doctors concerning terminology to cause great difficulties to the records subsystem. In addition, new knowledge tends to change the relationship of diseases to one another as well as to add new diseases. For this reason, medical records are coded; that is, a numeric code is assigned to each disease and trauma by a specially trained medical records librarian. The coding process involves a review of the working and final diagnoses and a study of the course of the illness. From these data a code is selected from one of the four commonly accepted coding schemes: the "Standard Nomenclature of Diseases and Operations," the "International Classification of Diseases," "Systematized Nomenclature of Pathology," and "Current Medical Terminology."

In addition to a disease indexing scheme, medical records are filed according to patient name, hospital identification number, surgical procedure, and attending or admitting physician. All of these schemes are based on numeric or alphanumeric codes. The hospital identification number is assigned by one of two distinct systems. Either a new number is given for every incident of hospitalization (the serial numbering system), or the same number is brought forward for all incidents of the same patient (the unit numbering system). Both systems have bad and good points. The unit system seems to be in ascension in the favor of most hospitals. All physicians are assigned numbers by the state in which they are licensed. We have referred to the operation numbering system above. These indices make the retrieval operation much simpler than it would be with no more than an alphabetic arrangement of records.

Reports and analyses on both a regular and exception basis are developed by the records subsystem. These include death rates, autopsy rates, average daily census, percentage of occupancy, average length of stay, and so forth. They involve retrievals from the files, using the indices appropriate to the report being developed. The reports divide generally into two classes: reports on individual patients, usually for internal use, and statistical studies for hospital management or medical audits.

Studies of the use and value of the records subsystem in many large hospitals show that information needs are not being met satisfactorily by current systems. We have alluded in a previous chapter to the increasing dependence on the hospital of outpatient and health screening services, home health care, and a more active part in community health interests. There is a corresponding increase in demand for greater community involvement in hospital affairs. This trend toward family-centered and community-centered medicine requires much more from the records subsystem than present methods can deliver. Comprehensive and systematic data must be maintained on the family as a unit and on the community as a whole. The usual hospital records department is ill-prepared for this task. Data on medical services performed by other agencies and institutions should be part of the patient's hospital record. This means efficient and timely exchange of information between facilities and agencies on a regular basis. Few such exchanges take place, and no standards are available for information interchange. Worse, no provision has been made in the record itself for these kinds of data if they were available. Such problems and the attendant requirements for standardization of terminology, uniformity of reporting formats and procedures, digital coding, and so forth, are clearly outside of our realm of influence here; but they are part of the future with which hospital data processing must cope. Metropolitan and regional medical records centers will be a fact, and the hospital information systems to be designed must account for them.

With the therapy system, we have reached the end of the input/output and data generation areas of the hospital. Virtually the entire range of data used or found in the hospital has been discussed, but nothing has been said about the methods of communicating these data from one system or subsystem to another. These interactions form the topic of the next chapter.

REFERENCES

American Hospital Association. *Reference Manual on Hospital Pharmacy.* Chicago, 1970.

"Innovations in Hospital Management." *Journal of the American Hospital Association,* vol. 43, no. 12 (1969).

Rourke, Anthony J. J. "Planning the Patient Space." *Journal of the American Hospital Association,* vol. 35, no. 4 (1961).

Scott, Wendell G., *Planning Guide for Radiologic Installations.* 2d ed. Baltimore: Williams and Wilkins, 1966.

Walter, Carl W. *The Aseptic Treatment of Wounds.* New York: The Macmillan Company, 1956.

7

The Communications System

INTRODUCTION

We have discussed information and data-processing functions—input, output, and internal processing—at great length in the previous chapters. We have made these functions the key to our examination of the hospital, viewing the entire institution as a system for collecting, generating, and disseminating information. Throughout all this, we have assumed that the reader understood what was meant by information and that he was familiar with communications concepts. We are about to begin a study of the hospital system most directly concerned with the handling of information. Perhaps at this point it is wise to examine some of the basic principles of information and communications before we proceed.

In the first section we will define some of the concepts and set the stage for our discussion of the communications system. The second section will specialize these concepts for the particular conditions of the hospital and also consider the input, output, and internal processing peculiar to the communications system. The chapter ends with an examination of the interactions and information transfers among the various systems and subsystems in the hospital.

INFORMATION AND COMMUNICATIONS

It has been shown that all information can be reduced to a series of binary digits, *bits* as coined by Tukey and Shannon, that is, to a stream of choices between zero and one. From this stream one may synthesize the most complex discrete symbols and then utilize the symbols or signals to convey any imaginable message. A message, in the sense intended here, is the communicable form of a concept, as opposed to its mental or semantic form; that is, a message is a set of symbols (a string of bits) that represents the concept in some conventional form agreed upon by the communicating parties.

In order to give these rather vague ideas some substance, consider the simplest model of a communications system. There are five basic elements—sender, transmitter, communications path, receiver, and recipient. The sender and recipient are persons or groups to whom the message is presumed to have meaning independent of the communications system. The transmitter is an encoding device that translates the message into a form appropriate to the communications path and initiates whatever action is required to introduce the translated message to the path. The translation process may involve much more than a change of form. Repetitions or redundancies may be added to increase the transmission reliability. Messages may be encoded or electronically scrambled to avoid unauthorized reception. The translation of a given symbol may depend upon previous symbols. Thus transmitters may have memories and other complex features aside from the encoding machinery.

Likewise, the receiver is more than a decoding mirror-image of the transmitter. The path may introduce undesirable symbols or change some symbols at random. These modifications of the message are known as noise. Reduction of noise is an important function of the receiver. By reducing noise, one can keep the level of error or ambiguity within acceptable limits.

The communications path is the method by which the message travels from the transmitter to the receiver. The accuracy of transmission, that is, the agreement between the encoded message from the transmitter and the encoded message delivered to the receiver, is a function of the path. Note that we are not concerned at this point with the agreement between the intended meaning of the sender and the interpreted meaning of the recipient. These semantic problems will be discussed a little later. We are concerned with the various parts of the communications path, the message structure and format, the message medium, and the set of procedures, operations, or mechanisms that move the message from the transmitter to the receiver.

As an example of the above system, consider one person talking to another. The sender formulates a message consisting of sounds that have conventional meaning. The lungs, throat, larynx, lips, teeth, and tongue translate the mental sounds into real sounds by expulsion of breath. The surrounding air carries the sound waves to the recipient's receiver, his ear. The ear decodes the arriving chain of pressure changes, which include the transmitted message along with a multitude of extraneous sounds, into a series of nerve impulses on the auditory nerve. The brain must then interpret these impulses and thus derive the message.

Clearly, a great many difficulties exist in communications, difficulties that must be overcome if messages are to be communicated successfully. These problems seem to exist at three distinct levels, technical, semantic, and influential. Technical problems of design of transmitters, receivers, and paths to achieve maximum accuracy of transmission have received the most attention and will preoccupy us in this treatment as well. They may not, however, be the most challenging. Semantic problems, the relationship between interpretation and intent, are much more complex. In fact, agreement between them can never be more than a tolerable approximation. Influential problems are concerned with the effectiveness with which the message leads to the desired conduct on the part of the recipient. This is the purpose of all communication and is the only provable, discernible effect of message reception.

These problems have deep significance for the whole area of language and meaning. Their solution, at least to the degree that meaningful communication can take place, is one of the most exciting areas of modern philosophic thought. Luckily, practice has not been required to wait for theory. Though the mechanisms are not clearly understood, it is clear that communication does take place, even among persons who have never heard of semantics. The requirements of space and purpose preclude any consideration of these topics in this text; so we also will be forced to muddle along, communicating with each other about communications without benefit of any real understanding of what we are doing.

The above statements might be interpreted to mean that the technical problems are devoid of philosophical significance, whereas the semantic and influential problems contain all of importance beyond the purely engineering design difficulties. Actually, some of the most elegant mathematics has been created to deal with the theory of information and its communication. No complete or definitive theory exists, but a great deal of work is being done, and some interesting results are available that seem to relate information to thermodynamics, Markov processes, and the statistical structure of language. We will refer to some of these results in what follows.

Communications systems of practical interest consist of a network of many sending and receiving units rather than one of each, as in our example. We would do well in what follows to restrict our definition of the communications system to exclude those elements that introduce the semantic and influential problems, the sender and the recipient of the message. We wish to extend the definition, on the other hand, to include the message structure within the system itself. Thus, our new definition of the communications system becomes "a network of transmitting units, receiving units, transmission paths, and message structures." Communications networks have two basic forms, centralized and decentralized. The decentralized network has a separate path from each unit to every other unit with which it must communicate. Centralized networks have one transmission path per unit, all connected to a central information clearing house or switching node through which all messages must travel on their way from the transmitter to the receiver. Centralized networks are used in computer-based information systems. The decentralized network is characteristic of inter-city telephone systems. Representative diagrams of these two types are shown in figure 7.1. Of course, it is possible to design systems using both types of network in some combination.

Communications systems also may be classified according to the type of transmitting and receiving units employed, the message structure involved, or the kind of transmission path used. The types of communications systems possible are almost endless. We shall see that hospitals utilize a great many different types.

Transmitting units and receiving units are usually the same unit physically, the distinction being a matter more of message direction. For our purposes, it is helpful to consider a single T/R unit capable of both transmitting and receiving, in some cases simultaneously. T/R units run from the most advanced electronic communications equipment to the simplest in/out tray for written notes. A great many unlikely things are used as paths for transmission of messages—all variety of paper and cardboard forms, marked with innumerable kinds of inked or carboned symbols, punched with different kinds of holes, or coded by many color schemes; electric wires in great abundance; audible coded signals; hand or body gestures; facial expressions; and so forth. The list is truly immense.

To each of these transmission paths there corresponds an appropriate message structure. One may characterize a system by describing how much of what kind of information must be sent from which T/R units to which other T/R units, how quickly, and how often—in other words, by the information flow pattern. These things help to determine the message structure. Several factors enter into such a description: (1) The number and distribution of T/R units, (2) the volume and flow rate of information, (3) transmission speed requirements, (4) reliability and accuracy requirements, and (5) loss, overload, and error penalties.

These factors are interrelated in a complex fashion. Raising the number of T/R units means increasing the transmission speed for the same information flow rate. High reliability usually reduces this speed, since many sophisticated steps must be taken in the transmission process. High penalty for error or loss demands repetition or redundancy, which, in turn, increases information volume. Allowances for transient system overload require more complex trans-mission methods or a larger number of message paths. The nature of these interactions, the trade-offs necessary to achieve the desired information collec-tion and dissemination within the other constraints of the system, must be specified before a successful communications system can be designed.

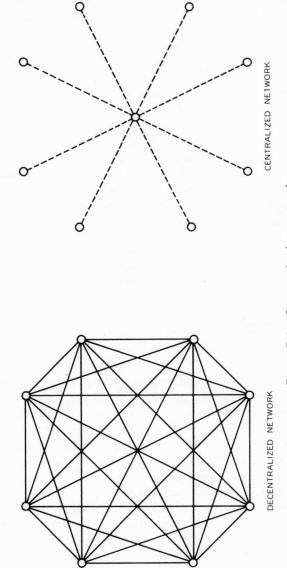

DECENTRALIZED NETWORK

CENTRALIZED NETWORK

Figure 7.1   Communications networks

115

These are, fundamentally, technical questions relating to the physics of message transmission in the system, that is, the nature of the medium and the T/R units. For example, the choice of pneumatic tube message transmission for all data of a certain type sets physical limits on transmission speed, information volume, and so forth. It is within these limits that the information theorist must work to design a message structure and T/R network that will meet the message transmission needs of the users.

One final word of importance in what follows: information and data are not synonymous. Data consist of any series of symbols transmitted or recorded. The symbols need not have meaning; or if they do, the meaning may not convey information. In its most general form, information is a collection of statements known to be true or false. Any proposition whose truth value is not either 0 or 1 contains no information. Communications principles may be used to convey data with or without meaning and with or without information content. We are concerned with the communications system of a hospital, where we shall find a great deal of communication with a small proportion of information transfer. This is a situation requiring correction where possible; but it must be remembered that much of human life, and therefore much of the goal structure of the hospital, concerns amenities and esthetics rather than information in the technical sense. Although these factors may be difficult to analyze, they must be accounted for and accommodated in the hospital communication system.

HOSPITAL COMMUNICATIONS

The principles outlined briefly in the previous section lead to deeper insights into the viewpoint we have adopted throughout the book of considering the hospital in terms of information handling. The concepts of input, output, and internal processing are analogous in some respects to the functions of the T/R units and transmission path. In one sense, we may say that input, as we have used the term, is the form of the message appropriate to acceptance by the transmitter portion of a T/R unit. Similarly, output is the form one would expect from the receiver portion. Internal processing, then, refers to the activities carried out by the transmission path in modifying the message.

This somewhat restricted view reduces all hospital systems to communications systems of one kind or another; that is, the only function of any information handling is its communication function. Clearly, storage is equally important, not to mention the use of information in decision making. There is also an implication inherent in this view that any information generated by internal processing activities must be considered noise, since communication is intended to move a message from transmitter to receiver without appreciable modification. We must look a little deeper for a fruitful analogy.

A possible refinement would be to add a T/R unit internal to each system and to allow processing between the reception of the input and the transmission of the output. This model would have the appearance shown in figure 7.2. It must be recognized that the input is being received from some other system and that the output is being transmitted to some other system. Further, we should distinguish between the system itself—consisting of a receiving unit, internal processing and storage equipment, and a transmitting unit—and the T/R units acting as communications interface with the rest of the hospital. There may be several of these, depending on system requirements and the nature of the message structure.

Finally, we shall choose to describe the communications system of the hospital as a centralized system, even though this may be inaccurate for some parts of the system as it presently operates. Thus, we arrive at the model shown in figure 7.3. The model has some validity, and we shall find it useful when we consider hospital intersystem communications.

The system we shall describe in chapter 9 has some of the characteristics of this centralized network. Another kind of refinement, used in that system, is called the "distributed" network. Instead of having one central node handling all message switching and storage tasks, one can distribute part of this load to a set

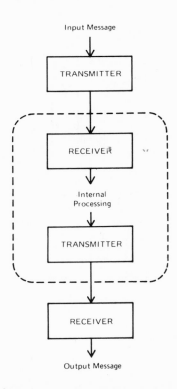

Figure 7.2   Hospital communications—preliminary model

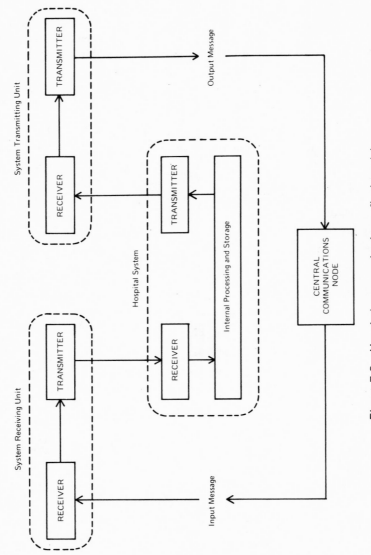

Figure 7.3   Hospital communications—final model

of subcentral nodes, retaining at the central node only those tasks and pieces of data likely to be required by some other hospital system. There are many economies to be gained by this approach, though the design of the total network may become much more complex. We shall leave our discussion of a system based on a quasi-distributed network to chapter 9.

Further refinements are possible. The central communications node of figure 7.3 is the heart of hospital communications and, as such, has many interesting features. Since only T/R units may transmit or receive messages, the central node must itself contain T/R units in sufficient numbers to handle the communications load. The central node performs certain internal processing functions, error checking and message switching, for example, so that fairly complex storage and processing equipment must be a part of its internal complement. We could attempt to produce a diagram showing a number of T/R units and internal processors, but the configuration is so dependent upon the system requirements that a generalized diagram would have little value.

In its simplest form, the central node would look very much like the model of any other hospital system in figure 7.3, with a transmitter, a receiver, and appropriate storage and processing gear. This similarity is the rationale for examining the communications system the same way we have the other hospital systems.

We have stated before in this text that the input to the communications system consists of the totality of messages sent or received in the hospital. To understand the implications of this, it is only necessary to recall the variety of message structures and the volume of data exchanged from all the systems and subsystems in the hospital. That means there must be an equal variety of receiver types capable of handling the volume expected. Further, all the intrasystemic communications must be considered. One way to reduce this hash to some kind of organization is to classify the input according to message type, source, and destination. We shall find this approach of value in the next section. For our purposes here, it is sufficient to recognize the complexity and magnitude of the problem.

Another interesting approach is to select a type of message and trace its path from first origin to final destination, recording all its stops along the way. One then proceeds to the next message type, and so on, until all types have been examined. This procedure has some associated difficulties in a hospital environment. There is a close correspondence between input and output, but not an exact one. Some systems generate a large proportion of the data transmitted and mix it liberally with input data. Many messages from one source go to several locations, often in slightly altered form for each. Other messages are combinations of information from many sources. This implies that the classification by source and destination must be a careful one, accounting for one-to-one, many-to-one, and one-to-many relationships. It would appear that these difficulties, although not insurmountable, make the first method a logical choice. It seems obvious that we must arrive at the same basic picture of the system by either method.

Before we attempt to classify messages, it is wise to recognize some inherent difficulties in the broad view we have taken concerning hospital communications. We are quite unable to treat the totality of hospital information transfer in a comprehensive and meaningful way. Fortunately, it is not necessary. For most of the input and output messages of importance to the data-processing functions of the hospital, there are fairly definite and well-defined structures. We may treat this subset of messages with some success. We have given a rather extensive discussion of message sources and destination in all the previous chapters. Everywhere we said "input," we may read "message destination"; and everywhere we said "output," we may read "message source." We have only to connect each input to its appropriate source or output to arrive at a reasonable approximation of a hospital information flow diagram. To complete the classification, we would have to label each message according to structure—discrete analog measurements, continuous physiological analog signals, decimal data, alphanumeric information, and so forth.

Internal processing in the communications system has three basic aspects, corresponding to the three functions of the central node. These are message verification, encoding-decoding, and message switching. Some messages require all these functions; others require only one or two. The determining factors are the complexity of the message and the requirements of the destination. In decentralized systems, without a central node, the communications path must perform these functions. If there is a requirement for complex processing, the centralized network has some obvious economic advantages.

There are many kinds of verification possible in a communications system. One could ascertain that a given message has the format required by the destination; this is called validity checking. One could determine that the data entered into the source transmitter have been received relatively error-free; this is called transmission accuracy checking. One could, by querying the sender, attempt to discover if the message sent reflects his intention; this is called verification, in the classical sense. Another sense of verification is vital in the hospital, that of authorization. Much of the information in the files should not be viewed by unauthorized individuals, nor should anyone but a physician order or prescribe for patients. In some cases, the recipient can be expected to verify authorization before taking the directed action, but this is best considered a central node responsibility. In any event, some action must be taken whenever a message cannot be verified or whenever an error is discovered. The action may involve correction of the error, retransmission, deletion of the message, or any other procedure that will eliminate the error or mitigate its consequences.

The encoding-decoding process is as varied as the message structures being transmitted. Conversion of data formats, for example, range from analog-to-digital conversion, with all the sampling and filtering procedures, to report formating, with headings, vertical and horizontal spacing, columnar breaks, and so forth. Many-to-one and one-to-many structures must be analyzed and new message structures built. The medium for some messages may change from transmission to reception. For example, a message entered by keyboard may be converted by the central node and displayed on a CRT. Again, a physiological condition recognized as critical may be transmitted as an alarm interrupt pulse and be received as a flashing light or buzzer. We refer to this type of processing as an encoding or decoding operation. The central node must be capable of a great variety of internal processing modes to accommodate the many kinds of message structures in the hospital.

Message switching is a kind of traffic control process. Messages of all sorts arrive at the receiving units of the central node. These messages must be sorted according to source and destination so that the appropriate encoding-decoding can take place. Some messages carry an originating address and a destination address. Others must be sorted by form and content. Occasionally, such factors as time of day, previous messages, or sender's authorization must be considered. After the encoding-decoding process, the message must be forwarded to its destination or destinations.

It should be clear that the central node is by far the most complex data-handling system in the hospital. In fact, every type of data processing done anywhere else in the hospital must be partially duplicated here to assure proper functioning of all the internal processing procedures. That is why we have been somewhat overgeneral and vague: to be explicit would repeat much of what has gone into the descriptions of the data-handling activities in the other systems. For example, in order to check the validity of a message requesting a prescription, the central node must verify, at a minimum, that the message originates with an authorized person, that the message is properly formated with all vital fields filled in, and that it is directed to the pharmacy. To do less would be to risk communicating nonsense over expensive equipment with great accuracy.

FLOW DIAGRAM PREPARATION AND INTERPRETATION

In the previous section we alluded to a simple method of arriving at an approximate information flow diagram for the hospital. We suggested in essence a connection of each input to a given system with the output of the system from which it originated. It comes to mind that this procedure is perhaps less simple than it sounds. In the next few pages we will go through the steps required to produce such a diagram and at the same time add a few enhancements that will make it a more useful document. We will utilize the results of the analysis in designing better methods of communicating information in the hospital. Because of our admitted inadequacy in the face of the total information flow, we will be somewhat restrictive, keeping our attention on the information related to data-processing activities.

The first step is the gathering of the inputs and outputs from each system and subsystem into a working table. These data are available from a quick perusal of the previous chapters. In a real situation, a careful survey would be made of the actual forms used, the messages sent, the conversations and discussions held, and the like, starting with the most important and voluminous messages and filling in detail as it becomes available. An example of this appears in figure 7.4. We have identified each category with a number for later reference. One output from central supply, the charge slips, is labeled 0/3-2, for the second output from the third system.

The next step is to attempt, for each input and output, to identify its source or destination. In some cases, these may be external to the hospital, or they may be original data from the patient. A partial listing of a table giving this kind of information is shown in figure 7.5. Note that we have used the previously assigned reference numbers to identify the inputs and outputs. Note also the use of *W, B,* and *P* to represent the added "systems" of external, building, and patient data sources or destinations. Including these pseudosystems assures that every input will have a source and every output a destination. Thus each entry in the input column will have a corresponding entry in the output column. This property may be used as a check on our efforts.

The final step is to prepare a diagram illustrating the relationships in figures 7.4 and 7.5. It is best at this stage to imagine a decentralized network; data transfers will be more meaningful. It is important to remember, however, that the hospital communications system has many aspects of a centralized network. The diagram that results might look something like figure 7.6.

In order to make the diagram more complete, we may repeat the three steps, adding more detail, breaking down the systems to subsystems, expanding the number and types of messages, and so forth. Figure 7.7 is an expanded version, including most of the message types mentioned in this text. It is possible to expand even further by considering other types of messages, but for our purposes the present diagram will suffice.

The value of diagrams like this is twofold: (1) A pictorial view should give new insights into the interactions and relationships among systems; (2) as we proceed with the design of an information communications system, the diagram should be helpful in focusing our attention on problem areas.

Let us point out some examples of these insights. First, it should be clear that there are many more message types than data types, which implies a great deal of redundancy and/or repetition. Some of this may be necessary to insure reliable message transmission, but the chances are good that at least some is the result of poor procedures. One of the major goals of an information communications system must be the elimination of all unnecessary redundant and repetitive data storage or transmission without appreciable loss of reliability.

Service System 1		Building System 2		Supply System 3		Therapy System 4		Management System 5	
Input	Output	Input	Output	Input	Output	Input	Output	Input	Output
Orders I/1–1	Performance O/1–1	Orders I/2–1	Performance O/2–1	Orders I/3–1	Performance O/3–1	Orders I/4–1	Performance O/4–1	Comments I/5–1	Orders O/5–1
		Sensor Data I2–2	Changes in Settings O/2–2	Requisitions I/3–2	Charge Data O/3–2	Patient Data I/4–2	Diagnoses O/4–2	Performance I/5–2	Public Relations Statements O/5–2
						Performance I/4–3	Instructions O/4–3	Charge Data I/5–3	Bills O/5–3
							Requisition O/4–4	Diagnoses I/5–4	

Figure 7.4   System input/output table

Input Label	Source	Output Label	Destination
I/1–1	O/5–1	O/1–1	I/5–2
I/2–1	O/5–1	O/2–1	I/5–2
I/2–2	O/B	O/2–2	I/B
I/3–1	O/5–1	O/3–1	I/5–2, I/4–3
I/3–2	O/4–4	O/3–2	.I/5–3
I/4–1	O/5–1	O/4–1	I/5–2
I/4–2	O/P	O/4–2	I/5–4, I/W
I/4–3	O/3–1	O/4–3	I/P
I/5–1	O/W	O/4–4	I/3–2
I/5–2	O/1–1, O/2–1 O/3–1, O/4–1	O/5–1	I/1–1, I/2–1 I/3–1, I/4–1
I/5–3	O/3–2	O/5–2	I/W
I/5–4	O/4–2	O/5–3	I/P

Figure 7.5   Correspondence of input and output

Secondly, the origins and destinations of most message types can be deduced from the form and content of the message itself. This means that a formal declaration of message destination is not required for effective communications. Economy of expression is one of the prerequisites of efficient system operation. To have this feature inherent in the system is indeed fortunate.

Thirdly, many of the messages have as their original source or final destination a storage area of some kind; that is, a large proportion of the message traffic in the hospital consists of entries to, or retrievals from, a data storage file. The implications of this fact for the information systems are enormous. For example, the centralization of the files would result, virtually in one step, in the centralization of a great deal of the communications system.

Insights of this kind can best be made by the systematic preparation and study of a flow diagram of the information and communication needs of the hospital as a whole, that is, of some form of figure 7.7.

THE ROLE OF COMMUNICATIONS

We stated previously that the communications system could be considered the nerve center of the modern hospital. This statement deserves amplification and support. Our discussions thus far have revolved around the internal goals of the

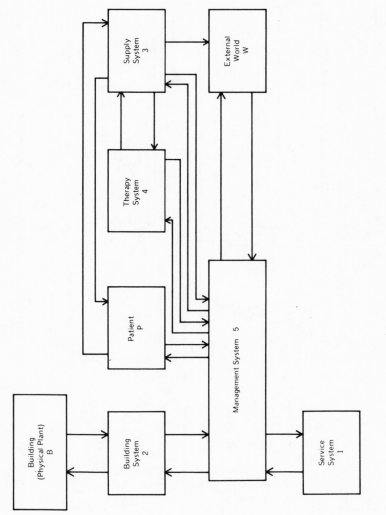

Figure 7.6   Preliminary diagram of data flow

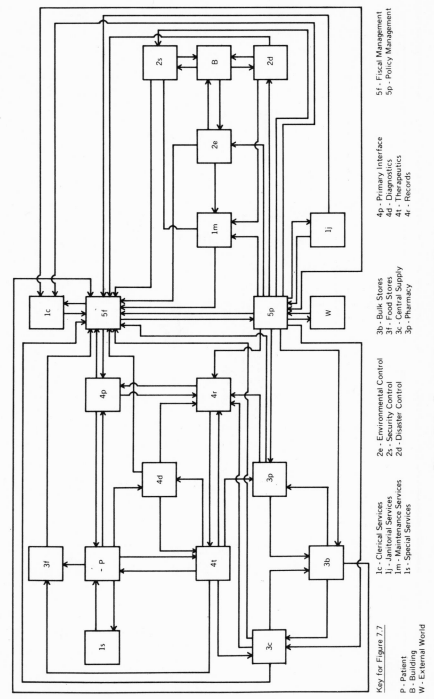

Figure 7.7   Expanded diagram of data flow

Key for Figure 7.7

1c - Clerical Services
1j - Janitorial Services
1m - Maintenance Services
1s - Special Services

2e - Environmental Control
2s - Security Control
2d - Disaster Control

3b - Bulk Stores
3f - Food Stores
3c - Central Supply
3p - Pharmacy

4p - Primary Interface
4d - Diagnostics
4t - Therapeutics
4r - Records

5f - Fiscal Management
5p - Policy Management

P - Patient
B - Building
W - External World

126

communications system and its input, output, and processing procedures. In this section we will investigate how the communications system fits into and accomplishes overall hospital goals.

The function of a communications network from the broad hospital viewpoint is twofold: (1) to collect, distribute, and store information in manners appropriate to the various operational modes of the hospital and (2) to integrate the operational activities and procedures into a coherent implementation of hospital policy. It is this latter function that concerns us here.

One of our examples of policy formation in chapter 5 was the development of a hospital budget. To have an effective budget, it was necessary to derive a consensus of the goals of the various special interest groups within the hospital. It was not clear just how this might be done, but communications played a significant role.

In our other example, the decision concerning computer purchase, a similar situation developed. It was essential that the decision satisify in some way the needs of both the medical staff and the administration and that both of these groups be willing to recommend and support the use of data processing.

These examples demonstrate one of the methods by which the separate activities of individuals, groups, and departments in the hospital are integrated into a coherent whole. Achieving consensus depends upon communication, not only of pieces of information, but also of attitude, status, intention, bargaining posture, perhaps even personality traits, all of which make up the environment of negotiation.

Another method of integration may be found in some of the technical imperfections of the communications system itself. This refers to the redundancy of many data paths in the hospital and the increased likelihood of data "leakage" through these paths. This results in a large amount of information concerning the activities of one area being propagated through other areas that have no specific need for the information. The phrase "rumor mill" is a recognition of this phenomenon.

There are times when the effects may be counterproductive, especially when they are directed toward personalities; but many times the effect is to provide an overall view of hospital operations that may be unavailable through normal channels. Thus the communications system may integrate hospital activities by providing data in unintended ways. Clearly, this is not the most desirable way to provide such data; but if data leakage is removed without a consideration for insuring broad general coverage of hospital activities, the results will be harmful.

Implementation of hospital policy has three important communications facets. First, the policy decision must be reached. Communications plays a large part in the decision process. Secondly, the decision must be distributed in an appropriate form to those responsible for its implementation. Finally, data concerning the progress of the realization of policy goals must be communicated back up the chain of authority.

Communications, then, appears in a vital role at each step in the implementation of hospital policy. Not only must each separate activity depend upon the input provided by the communications system for its internal operation; the coordination and control of the overall hospital functioning depend on communications also. This is the meaning of the phrase *hospital nerve center.* The message paths, storage methods, and T/R units integrate the hospital into an organic unity.

The above comments are necessarily idealized to some degree. Not every hospital has an effective communications network. But to the extent that the hospital is an organic unity with well-defined goals and an integrated plan of action—to that extent the hospital has an effective and well-tuned communications system.

The computer can play a most important role in the communications system. We will examine in chapter 9 what this role might be in a specific system design. It is well to caution the enthusiastic data-processing professional, however, that the computer can be only one part of a very complex and varied system. Much of the communications activity in a hospital is of necessity beyond the scope of data communications, and so it must remain.

8

Systems Analysis, Design and Implementation

INTRODUCTION

The purpose of the above chapters has been to introduce the concepts needed to design and develop effective computer systems for health care institutions. It seems axiomatic that good management should improve the quality and quantity of medical services and that good management depends on accurate and timely information. The computer can be instrumental in providing information more accurately and more quickly than manual methods. In this chapter we will attempt to provide some of the techniques and methods needed to support this thesis.

We believe the good computer system depends on good analysis; therefore, a considerable portion of the chapter will be devoted to a discussion of systems analysis techniques. For many readers this may be a review, but there are enough differences in the hospital environment to make the exercise valuable.

Following this, we will examine in some detail a few of the more prevalent types of commercially available hospital computer systems. This will not be a critical analysis, but rather a brief outline of the purpose, functions, and scope of the systems treated, intended more as a means of familiarizing the reader with current events. It should be noted that we are attempting to outline a broad field that is changing very rapidly, so that we will not aspire to anything like completeness. The best we can hope to do is to give a few instructive examples. There have been several detailed analyses of the many information systems on the market, performed by many people, each with his own orientation and motivation. A few are mentioned in the references at the end of the chapter.

THE SYSTEMS ANALYST IN THE HOSPITAL

Systems analysis is a powerful analytical tool for identifying and solving problems. The key word is *problems*. If the hospital had no problems, there would be no need for systems analysis. In chapter 2 we listed a few of the more pressing problems of data handling in the hospital. Of course, not all problems are of an information-processing nature. The hospital has many other types of problems, such as funding, personnel, organization, planning, and so forth, that have little direct connection with information processing. Systems analysis can be of value in isolating and attacking many of these problems also.

Our focus here will be on the application of systems analysis techniques to hospital EDP problems. This is not a new area of application, but much of the experience hospitals have had in the past has been less than happy. Many functions, especially in accounting, have been implemented successfully; but the total information-processing load of the hospital has been treated very infrequently. The author knows of no attempt along these lines that has met with unqualified success or that has been accepted by any significant number of hospitals. None of them are able to do the entire job, and many do what they do rather badly. They tend to dictate methods and procedures unacceptable to medical practitioners, and they often fail to provide the kind and quality of data needed by hospital management. Worst of all, the cost has been unreasonably high. At least part of the reason for the failure or qualified success of computer applications in hospitals is due to two basic factors: (1) the lack of understanding between data-processing professionals and hospital management concerning the nature of computers, the operation of hospitals, and the kinds of hospital problems EDP can address successfully and (2) the failure of system designers to distinguish between abstract solutions and real situations, that is, a failure to apply the fundamental principles of systems analysis.

The first of these factors will be alleviated as more and more computer specialists become involved with hospitals and as more and more hospital management and professional personnel become exposed to the concepts of data processing. The previous chapters of this text were intended to be a first move in the learning process. The following sections are designed to illustrate principles that will go a long way toward avoiding the second factor.

System Principles

The essence of systems analysis is methodology—a systematic approach to every problem utilizing proven principles. These principles are embodied in the following recommended five steps: environmental analysis, analysis by system, preliminary design, intermediate design, and system implementation.

Environmental Analysis. The hospital is an incredibly complex entity, but it is an entity, an interconnected whole. Changes in any part produce changes in others. Environmental analysis is designed to provide the facts concerning the total environment of the problem at hand and the likely impact of various possible solutions. The type of data needed will vary with the scope of the problem and the exact nature of the system proposed. Some items are important no matter what the conditions of the study. For example, the history of the hospital, its founders, and its growth is often of value in understanding its present circumstances. Of course, the organization, goals and objectives, and available resources are vital pieces of information for any study. The degree of automation and sophistication in all hospital areas gives meaning to the working environment and may be indicative of the kinds of solutions likely to be acceptable to hospital management. Not all of these data will be readily available to the systems analyst. He may have to do a lot of digging. Quite often, however, the value and significance of the information are proportional to the difficulty involved in obtaining it.

The aim of the analyst should be to learn enough about the hospital and its problems, and about hospital activities in general, to be able to converse intelligently on any hospital matter with the concerned personnel in the area. If he can achieve this kind of familiarity with the institution he is studying, the subsequent analysis will be that much more accurate and meaningful; and thus his recommendations will be that much more likely to be accepted.

There are three basic sources for the data needed in environmental analysis: reference materials, including documents of public record such as building permits and minutes of the area health planning council; the personal observations of the systems analyst; and hospital management, staff, and personnel. Background data can be obtained from any of the magazines and journals in this field, for example, *Hospitals, the Journal of the American Hospital Association, Modern Hospital,* the *Journal of the American Medical Association,* and the like. There is no substitute for direct personal observation, and the systems analyst should make it a habit to spend some time in all areas of the hospital as an unobtrusive observer. Many important facts concerning hospital problem areas can be obtained in no other way.

But by far the richest sources of information are the people working in the hospital. Discussions with administrative heads will reveal unstated goals and criteria for judging performance. Staff members, with their different emphasis, will provide other insights into operating conditions. Moreover, all personnel will have ideas concerning both the present and the proposed procedures, which the good analyst would do well to consider.

If hospital people are the best source of data, they are also very probably the least well utilized. Two methods are available for obtaining accurate and complete information from the management, staff, and personnel: the written questionnaire and the interview. The questionnaire should be used when the data needed are detailed and likely to require clerical effort or when it is not possible because of time or location to conduct personal interviews with the knowledgeable people in the area. Figure 8.1 is an example of a questionnaire designed for study of the radiology department of a medium-size community hospital. The questionnaire is directed at the possibility of automating the scheduling and film filing functions of that department, so that very specific kinds of questions are asked; however, it is a fairly good model for the development of more general questionnaires.

The questions presented in this survey will furnish a descriptive profile of your Radiology Department and will aid in defining problem areas. Please answer on separate sheets, preceding each answer with the question number.

A. General Information

1. What is the organizational structure of your department?

2. What percentage of inpatients have X rays?

3. What percentage of outpatients have X rays?

4. What types of X rays are most prevalent in the above areas?

5. What are the goals of the X-ray Department?

6. Have objectives been identified as steps in reaching these goals? Please list.

7. How many beds are included in the total hospital complex? How many will there be upon completion of any planned hospital expansion?

8. Approximately what percentage of the radiologist's time is consumed in standard X-ray procedures (chest, bone, GI, GU, etc.)?

9. Describe the teaching programs in practice in your department.

10. What is the annual growth rate within the Radiology Department in terms of patients and examinations?

11. What is the average length of stay within the hospital of the X-ray patient?

12. What would you list as primary problem areas within the department?

13. List secondary problem areas.

14. Are there any automation techniques presently being considered for use in scheduling, filing, reporting, etc., in the facility?

15. What increases in floor space (storage space, personnel working area, etc.) are being planned for the department?

16. Will new equipment be purchased? What types and what procedures are they capable of handling?

17. What data-processing facilities exist within the hospital (list equipment)? What hospital functions do they aid in handling?

18. Please furnish samples of all forms used in the X-ray process.

19. How many radiologists are there within the department?

B. Scheduling Information

1. At what locations within Radiology are scheduling functions performed? What types of exams are scheduled at each?

2. Which hospital areas (e.g., wards, etc.) and which clinic areas originate the greatest number of X-ray patients? What is this patient frequency? (Please estimate for each area.)

3. How many exams are scheduled at each scheduling area?

4. At what time during the day is patient scheduling activity the greatest?

5. Within what hours are exams scheduled?

6. What are the standard types of preexamination preparation for diagnostic X rays? Please list.

7. Which types of exams must be scheduled in advance?

8. How is the scheduling of special procedures handled?

9. If patient scheduling is considered as a "problem area," what are the specific "symptoms" associated with the problem?

10. Specifically, what patient and exam data are required during the scheduling process?

11. Are clinical comments on the patient's condition also used?

12. How are patients scheduled for standard diagnostic X-ray exams (time slot, time block, etc.)?

C. Film Filing Information

1. How many primary film filing areas are there? How many secondary areas? Which are located within the Radiology Department?

2. How are X-ray films transported to and from the filing areas?

3. How is the filing area notified of a pending scheduled X ray?

4. Is this procedure the same for all X rays?

5. How many films (or multiple film packets) are transferred (loaned out, transferred to other storage areas, used for current diagnosis) from each primary and secondary film storage area/day? Per week?

6. Are there peak periods of this activity? When are they?

7. How are these films monitored when outside their film area? How are they retrieved if needed for current diagnostic procedures?

8. Are patient data files maintained in the film file areas for use in locating film packets? For what other purpose are these patient data used?

9. How many patients are represented in each primary and secondary file area?

10. How are communications between these file areas maintained?

11. What are the current film folder loan-out procedures?

12. How frequently are films not available for current diagnosis because of loss, misplacement, inability to retrieve from "loaned-to" area promptly, etc.?

13. How are film folders coded? (e.g., terminal digit of patient unit no.)

14. Is there a separate X-ray accession number apart from the patient's hospital "unit number"?

15. How is this number used in the X-ray process?

16. If film filing is considered to be a problem area, what are the specific "symptoms" associated with the problem?

D. Reporting Information
  1. How many film viewing areas are there in Diagnostic Radiology?

  2. How many more are planned?

  3. How many dictaphones are in each area?

  4. How many transcribing machines are there?

  5. How many films are read in one average day by a radiologist? (If there are great differences due to exam or procedure type, please indicate.)

  6. Approximately what percentage of all diagnostic X-ray procedures are represented by "negative" or "no change" reports?

  7. Are all or some diagnostic X rays indexed or coded for the purpose of future retrieval and use?

  8. What are these uses?

  9. What percentage of all X-ray cases are so coded?

 10. What coding or indexing methods are used?

 11. Is this method used and accepted by *all* the department's radiologists?

 12. What are the report review and sign-off requirements within the department?

 13. Where and how are reports sent when finally approved?

 14. What type of dictating systems are used in the reporting of X-ray results?

 15. Is the Nyematic system being considered for present or future use for report dictation? For use elsewhere in Radiology?

 16. Approximately what percentage of the diagnostic report requests come from each of the hospital originating areas? Do you expect this to change in the existing or planned facility?

 17. What type of fixed patient descriptor data is used in generating an X-ray report? From what source is it obtained?

 18. If reporting is considered to be a problem area, what are the specific "symptoms" associated with the problem?

 19. Are there hours of peak activity during the day for report dictation? What are they?

Thank you for your kind assistance in this study.

Figure 8.1   Sample radiology questionnaire

Whenever practical, the interview remains the most effective way of gathering facts. A good interview technique is a skill that must be developed by anyone with ambitions in systems analysis. This is particularly true in the sensitive areas of a hospital. The previous chapters have stressed the differences in goals, outlook, and interest of the various groups in the hospital. The skilled interviewer will recognize these facts and guide the interview in the direction that will establish rapport with the person being interviewed, and he will thus attain the goals of the interview.

There are three types of systems interview: the initial or introductory interview, the fact-gathering interview, and the follow-on or clarification interview. The purposes of the introductory interview are to sell the personality of the systems analyst as a sympathetic and competent listener and to explain the objectives of the study and the advantages hoped to be gained for the person being interviewed. The initial interview should be used to get a reading on the respondent's attitudes and interests and to set the stage for the second phase of discussions.

The approach and strategy suggested by the introductory interview are followed in the fact-gathering interview. The most vital point to remember in planning this kind of interview is to be prepared, to know enough about the respondent's area and interests to talk to him intelligently. The analyst should have well in mind the questions he wants answered. As the interview proceeds, the respondent will provide information that the interviewer should record later for use. One of the skills needed by a good systems interviewer is effective note-taking. He should learn to take sufficient notes to be able to reconstruct significant parts of the discussion. Equally important, the interviewer must be sensitive to the moods of the respondent, particularly signs of tiring, and end the interview short of losing the confidence and rapport built up in the introductory interview.

Some time later, after the data gathered have been analyzed, a follow-on interview may be necessary to fill in gaps or clarify questions that arise in the evaluation. Usually, the follow-on is short and to the point, designed to answer specific questions. Another use of this type of interview is to try out new ideas on the people who will be most affected.

The results of all reference studies, questionnaires, and interviews should be collected and summarized in a single project file for use in the design phase.

Analysis by System.   The second step in the systems analysis of a hospital is to study the logical divisions of the particular institution in much the same way that we have studied the general hospital in this text. Building upon the framework of system breakdown given here, we can fill out the meat of the skeleton with specific details of the case at hand. Flow diagrams, both of materials and information, should be made for the hospital as a whole and then for each system and subsystem. The diagrams in chapter 7 may act as models. The more complete and detailed these drawings are, the clearer will be the understanding of the system relationships and functional operation of the hospital. Added to the documentation of the environmental analysis, this system view will provide the basis for the design of the information system.

It may be that only a portion of the hospital is being considered or studied. In this case, the amount of detail needed for peripheral areas will be reduced; however, some data should be collected, since there will be effects on all areas owing to the system being designed. In addition, if other areas become subjects for later studies, the materials collected now will be of value.

Preliminary Design.   The preliminary design is the third step in the logical process of system design. The purpose is to create a model of the hospital, or at least of the portion being automated, in terms of data-processing operations, but without regard to the method for accomplishing them. The systems analyst is not concerned with the type of computer system involved; indeed, at this point it has not been decided that a computer will be used. He is concerned with inputs, outputs, and internal processing functions.

One further detail is added in this phase of the design, the contents, and the size and structure of the data storage files needed to support all information-processing functions. These files may be tapes or disks, or a simple bulletin board. The medium is not important here. What is important is that data be classified into logical groups, that the content reflect all necessary information, and that the capacity of the files be sufficient for the data storage requirements.

These system features—input, output, and processing functions and file support—are put together into a preliminary information flow system. Much of this system may be identical with present processing methods. Other parts will contain changes in traditional methods or completely new functions recognized in the analysis. This preliminary design is used as a check on the previous steps. If more facts are needed, if there are inefficiencies in the data-handling methods, or if inconsistencies exist in the information provided by hospital personnel, they will show up in the preliminary design model. The design is then modified to reflect the true situation.

When a preliminary design has been developed that seems to incorporate the best of current methods and the recommendations of the systems analyst, management can be presented with the proposed new system. This usually means administrative heads and top-level medical staff as well as the board of directors. Since the preliminary design is in functional terms rather than technical EDP concepts, hospital management should find no difficulty grasping the intentions of the new system. Indeed, it is the job of the analyst to insure that there is no confusion or misunderstanding.

Intermediate Design.   Using the preliminary design materials as approved by management, the systems analyst now proceeds to develop the working system design; that is, he adds detailed data-processing steps and operating sequences to the broad functional blocks of the preliminary design. He also chooses the method—manual, mechanical, or electronic—for each function. Many factors must be considered in deciding on the details of the system. The analyst must be knowledgeable about computer hardware and other types of information-handling equipment. He must be familiar with the forms and procedures of manual data processing. He must be aware of the many techniques for handling files. Finally, he must be creative in utilizing his knowledge and the hospital's resources to develop the most cost-effective system that will meet the processing requirements agreed upon by management.

The various parts of the intermediate design must be specified in sufficient detail that the people who will implement these parts, the forms analysts, electronic engineers, programmers, and so forth, can work directly from the design specifications. Of course, this is not a final system design, since many changes may occur during implementation. The final design will be embodied in the procedures manual, operations manual, and system manual, which make up the final system documentation.

System Implementation. The last step in systems analysis is the actual implementation of the system design. This is no more than a careful overseeing of the work of the people responsible for following the instructions of the intermediate design specifications.

There is a dangerous tendency among EDP professionals to produce a system with low stability, that is, one in which nearly every element is going through continuous "improvement." New products and methods come to light daily, and the desire to incorporate the attractive ones into a partially implemented system can be irresistible. But this impulse must be resisted. Nothing is as destructive of morale as the discovery that yesterday's established design is today's discard in favor of a "better way." Freezing the system design allows for the most efficient use of resources and at the same time maintains the confidence of the hospital and data-processing personnel.

Planning

All of the above five steps depend on an effective plan of action. Planning is itself a topic worthy of careful consideration; its general principles are applicable in many areas. In creating a data-processing installation for a hospital, a plan is absolutely indispensable. It is worth a little of our time here to review some of the principles of planning, especially as they relate to system design and implementation.

The word *planning* is used rather loosely to describe a great variety of dissimilar activities. The process to be considered here must be separated sharply from those activities, also called planning, that do not follow the principles and do not produce the results that are effective in guiding future decisions. We will discuss that variety of planning that involves a substantial *change* in present circumstances. Thus, the creation of a budget for a continuing project or organization, without consideration of alternatives to current policies, does not qualify as planning. We must exclude also activities not intended to be a guide for concrete future activities. Such academic exercises, foredoomed to lie dormant on the planners' desks, have little to teach us. Their fate is usually known in advance and creates its own attitude and approach in the minds and actions of those involved.

We are talking, then, about a set of activities aimed at determining guidelines for concrete changes in the structure, organization, or procedures of an institution or some system thereof. We may take the foregoing sentence as our definition of planning.

In the progress of his activities, the planner, in our case the systems analyst, will find himself involved in an iterative process that is basic to the kind of planning for change of interest to us here. Souder, Clark, Elkind, and Brown originated a conceptual model of this iterative process in a Public Health Service research project. In their model, the process has three distinct phases: investigation, synthesis, and evaluation. Though the model was created for hospital planning, it has validity outside that restriction. It seems clear that any plan will begin with an investigation of the requirements implied by the goals and of the resources available to meet them. When sufficient facts are thought to be at hand, the planner will likely set down a tentative arrangement or allocation of resources to satisfy the goals. This synthesis phase is followed by an evaluation of the proposed scheme with respect to desired results. It may be that important elements of the problem have been disregarded, requiring further synthesis. This may be thwarted by a lack of facts, requiring further investigation, and so forth. A complex planning problem is composed of many projects, each of which follows the iterative process. Thus, it is likely that investigation of one project will be concurrent with synthesis of another and evaluation of still another. It also may happen that the synthesis phase will produce several alternatives that require examination, so that a given project in the overall plan may have several optional schemes, all in different phases of the planning process.

Successful planning is not an accident. It is composed of specific ingredients, the planning principles we mentioned above. They may be codified into six laws of effective planning: specify planning goals, outline steps to be followed, analyze the current situation, set a time schedule, assign project responsibilities, and review at predetermined stages.

Specify Planning Goals. An effective plan is a guide to action. It should be directed toward creation of, or change in, a structure, procedure, or system. But changes must be directed, meaningful, goal-oriented. Without goals, change is mere reaction or aimless motion. The goals must be specific, practical, realistic. The more clearly and completely these goals are specified, the more likely they are to be realized.

Outline Steps to be Followed. Again, a plan must be action-oriented.

There must be a concrete series of steps leading to the realization of each goal. These steps become a kind of road map, directing energies and resources where needed.

Analyze the Current Situation. It is often surprising to high-level management how little they know about the operation of their organization. A study of current systems and procedures should be a standard part of the investigation phase of each step in the planning process. Before changes are implemented, the present conditions must be known and understood.

Set a Time Schedule. Effective planning always involves carefully defined completion dates for each major element of the system. It should be emphasized that unrealistic deadlines can be as bad as no deadlines. Sufficient time must be allowed for adequate completion of key elements; otherwise, schedules will suffer.

Assign Project Responsibilities. Each element or project directed toward the realization of each step in the plan must be the express responsibility of an individual. This individual must have authority to perform his duties adequately.

Review at Predetermined Stages. Each step of the implementation schedule should be evaluated at regular intervals to insure that deadlines are being met, that goals are still valued, and that corresponding or complementary projects are proceeding as desired. A final review as each step is completed and a total project review when all steps are completed should ascertain if the goals have been met as planned.

The reader should compare these planning principles with the systems analysis steps listed previously. We have on the one hand: (1) environmental analysis, (2) analysis by system, (3) preliminary design, (4) intermediate design, and (5) system implementation; and on the other: (1) goals, (2) action steps, (3) current analysis, (4) schedule, (5) responsibilities, and (6) review.

The similarities are striking. The systems analyst may follow either or both of these sets of proscriptions in his endeavors. The point, as we stated at the beginning of the chapter, is that some systematic rules should be followed to insure that all factors are considered. The rules are meant to be guides to successful systems analysis and design. It must be admitted that no set of suggestions offers a complete guarantee of success; therefore, a few comments by way of disclaimer are in order.

The best plan may fail. This is the proverbial effect of unpredictable events, the basic raw materials of planning. The converse, of course, is that the worst plan may succeed. Good planning should minimize the probability that unexpected events will doom the plan to failure. A review of the successes, and the failures, of large hospital information systems projects should instill some healthy humility in the minds of systems analysts.

The very act of studying an organization, formulating a plan to achieve system goals, and evaluating the plan in the light of changing circumstances, has an enormous effect on an institution, even though the plan itself may never be implemented. Many organizations have discovered that the systems analysis and design needed to install a new computer system have uncovered vast ineffi- ciencies and wasted effort in the current manual system that were heretofore unsuspected. Often the elimination of these poor procedures and the substitu- tion of effective management controls made the proposed computer system unnecessary.

The reasons for this are partly technical and partly psychological. All systems become obsolete in time. Good design can extend system life, allowing the system to grow with the organization, up to a point. Eventually, it must be discarded or it becomes counterproductive. In addition, the principle of self-ful- fillment operates here. The involvement of people in the decision-making process tends to improve attitude and work habits, thus increasing productivity. This does not imply that any plan is as effective as a good plan. Attitudes that are not reinforced by reality will decay rapidly. A poor plan is probably more effective in this sense than no plan at all, but the most effective one will set realistic goals, consider the needs of the individuals in the organization, and maintain a receptive attitude to changes in the progress of the plan. The point is that all major planning activities tend to affect their subject in major ways.

We may summarize the above comments as follows: Systems analysis and general planning have many points in common, perhaps the most important of which is the need for a systematic step-by-step approach. Following these principles does not guarantee success, but it is the best we can do. It seems clear that the systems analyst who is armed with good methods has a better chance of creating effective and successful systems.

CURRENT HOSPITAL SYSTEMS

The computer systems currently available from computer manufacturers, hos- pital associations, and service bureaus may be classified as business information systems, medical or "total" information systems, and special systems. In this section we will give some examples of each, a brief description of a representa- tive member, and some of the advantages and disadvantages. Let me repeat that no claim is made here for completeness or in-depth analysis. We are giving a few examples of commercially available systems as a way of leading into a discussion of the author's suggestions for a new approach to the problem. The interested reader may obtain more details from the vendors of the various systems. The examples selected were chosen because of the author's familiarity with them rather than because of any inherent superiority in them. It will become obvious that no endorsement is intended.

Business Information Systems

Historically, computers first entered the hospital as aids in the routine clerical activities associated with hospital accounting. The success of EDP in the business world and the orientation of hospital accountants toward automated business methods made this a natural step. Computers are still being used in this way in the overwhelming majority of hospitals using computers.

The business systems occur in two distinct types, the stand-alone system, requiring the hospital to have its own computer, and the shared system, in which several hospitals utilize the same equipment on a batch or partially on-line basis. In a number of hospitals, the shared systems far outweigh the single systems.

Shared hospital accounting systems are available from at least three manufacturers: International Business Machines, Honeywell Information Systems, and Burroughs, with the possibility of late entries by National Cash Register and Control Data. Single systems are supplied by virtually all computer hardware vendors. The hospital can obtain the services of a computer-sharing organization in many ways. Several service bureaus have arisen in the past few years to serve this market, notably Shared Medical Systems, Compucare, and Tel-Data. In addition, many of the Blue Cross and other hospital associations across the country have installed computer equipment and are providing shared accounting as one of their services to hospitals.

We will describe one of the systems in common use, the Hospital Computer Sharing System (HCSS), supplied by Honeywell. The similarities between HCSS, IBM's SHAS, Burrough's BHAS, and others are much greater than the differences. Details of hardware and procedures vary; but the intent, function, and merits are almost identical.

HCSS consists of nine related systems designed to perform most of the routine clerical tasks usually assigned to the hospital business office. They are: patient accounting, general ledger/responsibility reporting, cost allocation, inventory reporting, property ledger, accounts payable, personnel records, payroll, and preventive maintenance.

Patient Accounting. Patient accounting offers data input editing, automatic charge description and pricing for most items, posting of charges to patient and departmental accounts, automatic insurance apportionment, billing, and complete accounts receivable aging and control.

General Ledger/Responsibility Reporting. The general ledger/responsibility reporting system provides a uniform framework for reporting and controlling hospital costs and revenues that is based on the AHA Chart of Accounts for Hospitals. It also provides assistance in budget preparation.

Cost Allocation. Cost allocation consists of allocation of allowable operating costs among the various hospital cost centers on the basis of floor space, nursing hours, laundry usage, and so forth, for use in obtaining medicare reimbursement.

Inventory Reporting. Inventory reporting provides summary reports on current stock balance, on-order quantities, reorder points, safety stock levels, and so forth, which can be used for inventory forecasts and for calculating economic order quantities and times.

Property Ledger. The property ledger system is designed to supply the information necessary for the effective management of the physical assets of the hospital. Calculations of depreciation, reimbursement levels, optimum insurance coverage, and the like, are part of the system.

Accounts Payable. Accounts payable handles vendor invoices, patient refunds, utility bills, service contracts, insurance premiums, tax payments, and so forth. It provides input to the general ledger system.

Personnel Records. The personnel records system provides information for performance reviews, wage and salary evaluations, and benefit programs. Management reports on terminations, hires, job title changes, and so forth, and federal reports such as minority and wage and hour reports are part of the system.

Payroll. Complete processing of paychecks for both hourly and salaried employees is provided by this system, as well as monthly and annual reports.

Preventive Maintenance. The routine scheduling duties associated with the maintenance of major equipment in the hospital is performed by successive sorting and printing of work lists, instructions, and maintenance scheduled.

The hardware configuration required for the communications version of HCSS consists of the following:

Communications processor	Series 200 computer with 28K memory 1 Magnetic tape 1 Magnetic drum 1 Communications controller
Batch processor	Series 200 computer with 49K memory 6 Magnetic tapes 1 Line printer 1 Card reader

The system will support as many as 20 small hospitals, and there seems to be no practical limit to the number of beds that can be put on the system.

Input for most functions is by teletype, the transactions being recorded on the drum of the communications processor. Reports, except for a few such as the demand summary bill and daily census, are produced in batch mode on the batch processor. The reports are then delivered to the hospitals by truck.

There are many advantages in the use of shared business systems such as HCSS. Among those claimed by Honeywell are: the availability of better equipment and personnel, a broader base of comparative information for decision making, reduction in cost and time of implementation, and the sharing of costs among many institutions. We might add two advantages often not mentioned by the manufacturers. First, a shared business system allows a hospital to try data processing with low risk and a small initial investment; if the hospital finds the costs too high or the procedures not amenable to its operating philosophy, there is not a heavy penalty involved in a change of decision. Secondly, a large central facility provides a career path for data-processing professionals that the hospital can never match. Thus, the turnover in high-level EDP management will likely be lower. If one considers the costs of executive replacement, this is not an inconsiderable factor.

There are also some significant disadvantages to the shared approach. Flexibility is extremely low; the systems implemented must be a joint decision of all sharing institutions. A further implication is that control over operating policy, funding levels, personnel, priorities, and so forth, must be shared also. For many hospitals, this is an unacceptable constraint. Stability of the EDP facility is difficult to insure, especially if a commercial service bureau is involved. But perhaps the most serious disadvantage, especially for the medium-sized, progressive hospital, is that the shared facility solves only one small portion of the information-processing needs we have identified. The recognition of this fact has led to the more ambitious automation projects known as "total" information systems.

Medical Information Systems

Many studies have been made of the communications and data-handling tasks of the hospital. Whenever these studies have attempted to be comprehensive in scope and truly palliative in intent, the result has been called a "total information system." Three features seem characteristic of these attempts:

1. The system tries to do everything for everyone in the hospital.
2. Nothing can be done (within the scope of system tasks) without going through the system.
3. Extensive, in fact, almost exclusive, use is made of electronic terminals, storage devices, and computer methods in general.

The system requirements as they have been developed seem to demand these characteristics.

Several systems of this type have been built for specific institutions, with no intention of developing a marketable product. The various systems of Massachusetts General Hospital are examples, as are the projects at the University of Missouri Medical School, Kaiser Foundation Hospital in Oakland, and the Latter Day Saints Hospital in Salt Lake City. An examination of these systems can be very instructive. It is highly recommended for the analyst who is seriously considering work in this area.

Other systems of the "total" variety have been designed with the hospital marketplace in mind. These include the systems being sold by Spectra Medical Systems, Technicon, Biomedical Computer Services, Sanders, and National Data Communications, Inc. of Dallas. As in the case of business systems, the competing systems are sufficiently alike to make it unnecessary for our purposes to discuss all of them. We will examine the REACH system.

REACH, an acronym for real-time electronic access communications for hospitals, was designed by National Data Communications, Incorporated, in conjunction with a community hospital in Texas and the systems staff of the computer hardware vendor. It is completely proprietary and never sold in source form. The system is for lease only. NDC contracts to do any programming, hardware, or procedural changes needed in the system; the customer is not allowed to modify anything. On the other hand, sufficient flexibility is claimed to make extensive modifications unnecessary.

The hardware for REACH is of three types: I/O terminals, local communications processors, and remote heavy duty processors. The terminals were designed and built to NDC specifications by Raytheon. We will examine them more closely a little later, when we discuss system operation. The communications processor is a small word-oriented minicomputer with associated mass storage equipment. Its main function is to control terminal operations, store local data for rapid access, and communicate transactions to the central facility. The central facility operates in many ways like the shared business system computer, performing the basic accounting functions and heavy record storage tasks.

One of the most interesting features of REACH is its dedication to extreme reliability. It is claimed that REACH is a zero-downtime system, and the experience so far indicates at least a close approximation is achieved. This is accomplished by duplicating virtually every piece of hardware and connecting everything together with electronic switches; that is, there are two communications processors and two mass storage devices, all interconnected and all operating simultaneously on the same data. If any one of these machines has a problem, its twin can carry on independently. Of course, if both processors are down, the system dies; but this is rather unlikely. There are also two computers at the central facility, thus assuring virtually trouble-free operation.

Another unique feature of REACH is the large amount of personnel support included as part of the service. It includes technical personnel for installation, software customizing, and equipment maintenance and education specialists to train the administrative, professional, and clerical staff in all aspects of usage and operation of the system.

System operation has many aspects in common with the other commercial entries in the field. Let us examine the terminals first. They were designed and build by Raytheon to REACH specifications, and for some time were unavailable for general sale. Raytheon has been marketing a version of the terminal recently under the name *Pulse*. It consists of a standard CRT display and keyboard with two rather unique features, a badge reader for operator identification and a series of line selector buttons along the left margin.

It is this last feature that characterizes the REACH system. Operation may be illustrated by describing the procedure by which a physician orders a prescription for one of his patients.

1. The first action for any terminal operation consists of inserting the user's badge in the badge reader. The badge identifies the user, specifies his level of authorization, and enables the terminal.
2. The terminal responds to the insertion of a physician's badge with a list of the patients in the hospital admitted by or being cared for by this doctor. If a nurse inserts her badge, she is presented with a list of the patients on her ward. The doctor selects one of the patients by pressing the button next to his name. (If the doctor has more than 20 patients, he may view the next "page" by entering "NEXT" on the keyboard.)
3. The screen then displays a list of options to be selected, such as laboratory test, X ray, special diet, or pharmacy. The physician selects the pharmacy button.
4. Subsequent displays allow the doctor to select either generic or trade names for drugs or to order them alphabetically; to specify the dosage and frequency; and to view the finished prescription before releasing it for communication to the pharmacy.
5. The doctor may then return to the list of options or his patient roster, or sign off, removing his badge and thus disabling the terminal.

A similar operating procedure is followed by the nursing staff, admissions clerks, technicians, and all other hospital personnel interacting with the system. Each hospital data input or output function has a set of displays and an associated tree structure of options designed to capture all orders, convey all messages, and store all relevant information within the scope of the system. The REACH promotional material makes a point of stressing that paperwork is gone forever.

In addition to being a communications system, REACH attempts to be an administrative tool. Many of the features of the shared accounting system may be found in the central utility concept of REACH. The difference is in the means of data capture. Most shared business systems utilize manual entry of charge slips as a distinct procedure in the operation of the system. REACH captures the *order* of a chargeable item and thereby records the *charge* connected to the delivery of the item automatically. Reports, in the few instances where voluminous output is mandatory, are produced by high-speed printers at the hospital.

All the advantages claimed by other types of shared facility are claimed by the REACH system. In addition, REACH has the potential of reducing lost and late charges, ordering and delivery errors, and clerical work load on professional personnel.

There are three major areas of doubt concerning REACH and similar systems on the part of hospital administration, nursing staff, and physicians. The first of these is cost: REACH costs between six and seven dollars per patient-day. In all fairness, competitors offering comparable services are priced in the same range as REACH. Clearly, hospitals must decide if this type of system justifies the expense and if part of the cost can be passed on to the patient or his guarantor.

Another question of importance is the likelihood of physician and nurse acceptance. The field is too new for any real certainty, but reports to date are not encouraging. The problem is one of education and orientation, perhaps requiring the growth of new teaching methods in medical schools over a period of years. The vendors of these systems cannot be blamed for creating the problem. However, the doctor-computer interaction may tend to exacerbate the situation. This, at least, is one of the concerns of some hospital administrators when considering the purchase of a total information system.

Finally, an area of very real concern is the degree of dependence the hospital must place upon an unproved device under the operating conditions of a total system. Because it is a complete system, because paperwork disappears, and because all orders are placed through the computer, the difficulties faced by the hospital if the system goes down approach catastrophic proportions. This is a very unlikely event, but unlikely events are daily fare in an institution built to handle crises in human health. When it happens, the hospital is crippled. No other single piece of equipment or apparatus could so totally disable the hospital. There is little wonder that hospital management has been hesitant to trade their current problems for these new ones.

Special Systems

There are a variety of applications in the hospital that have been implemented on special-purpose, dedicated equipment. These include research-oriented data acquisition systems, patient monitoring systems, automated medical history taking, and clinical laboratory systems.

Of these special applications, clinical laboratory automation has received the most attention from commercial vendors. Four of these, B-D Spear, Berkeley

Scientific, Digital Numeric Applications, and Digital Equipment Corporation, have installed virtually all of the fully supported systems installed today. IBM supports hardware and operating systems software only, leaving application program responsibility to the user. A few other firms have indicated plans to produce a complete laboratory system, but the above companies seem to have the largest share of the market well in hand.

We will examine the *Clindata* system of Berkeley Scientific Laboratories. BSL was formed in 1965 for the specific purpose of developing and marketing clinical laboratory systems. There are many BSL systems installed, with several more in various stages of implementation.

The hardware for Clindata consists of the following:

PDP-8/L Central processor (8K to 20K)
Magnetic disk
Magnetic tape
Teletype or CRT channel (up to 16)
Digital data channel (up to 28)
Analog data channel (up to 19)
Line printer
Card reader
Special data input consoles

One of the most interesting features of the Clindata system are the special consoles. These are BSL-designed data input terminals for use by lab technicians rather than clerk-typists. Test-specific terminals for Coulter S, urinalysis, electrophoresis, bacteriology, differential counts, and morphology are provided, along with a general purpose terminal. Data entry by the technician has many good and bad features. Many users, both BSL and others, swear by it, while some labs claim it is more economical and faster to train special data entry clerks. The final decision on the merits of this method awaits a definitive study by an objective body.

It should be clear from our previous discussion of the clinical laboratory that a computerized information system, to be truly beneficial to the hospital and the laboratory, must reduce errors or reduce clerical work load. The Clindata system claims to do both. This is accomplished by maintaining three general classes of data: patient admissions data, test request data, and test result data. In addition, billing information, communications with the dietary and pharmacy areas, and medical records reports are handled by the BSL system.

Entry of admissions and test request data is by keyboard, either teletype or CRT. A library of 500 tests may be selected. These entries are in conversational mode, with considerable editing and checking throughout, under control of a sophisticated system monitor. Admission and test entry routines require about 30 seconds per patient with experienced operators. Mark sensing of cards for test request entry is also available, though no operational system is so equipped as yet. Test result entry is by special console, keyboard, or mark sense. For a few instruments, direct on-line analog entry is available, though special hardware and software options called Chemdata are required.

The output consists of a variety of printed reports utilized by admissions, billing, the physician, the ward nurse, the lab technicians, and laboratory management. A partial list follows:

Directory of admissions
Directory of specimens
Test summary report
Master work sheet
Individual work sheet
Collection list
Automated instrument load list
Individual report (normal or query)
Ward report
Cumulative report

The general flow of data and samples through the laboratory using Clindata is as follows:

> A list of admitted patients is sent to the laboratory once each day for entry into the computer. Throughout the day, test requests are received from the wards and entered into the system. Before the morning collection rounds, a drawing list and sample labels are printed. The specimens are drawn and returned to the lab with identifying labels. They are distributed to the work stations according to the master work sheet. Individual sheets are waiting at the stations, where they are matched with the specimens and the tests performed. Test result data are entered and the identification verified by the computer. As patient series are completed, reports are printed and distributed to the wards. Special reports for billing and cumulative results are printed at night.

The advantages claimed by BSL for its Clindata system seem to be realized to a large degree in installations that have done a good job of implementation, using competent people and having high-level management involvement. The most serious challenge to this record is in the area of hardware reliability and maintenance service. There seems to be user consensus that result reporting has been speeded up, errors reduced, and utilization of laboratory personnel increased where Clindata has been installed. It has been reported that the BSL competitors have had similar user reactions in most of their installations.

They also have had similar complaints. Among these are lack of hardware and software maintenance in remote areas, overstatement of advantages and savings, and understatement of the level of technical computer competence required by laboratory personnel.

REFERENCES

Clinical Laboratory Computer Systems. J. Lloyd Johnson: Northbrook, Ill., 1971.

Garrett, Raymon D.; Levine, Arnold; and O'Neil, Roy. *Visual Input/Output Devices for Hospital Information Systems.* New Orleans: Tulane University Press, 1969.

Encyclopaedia Britannica, Inc. *Handbook of Biomedical Information Systems.* Chicago, 1971.

Krieg, Arthur F.; Johnson, Thomas J.; McDonald, Clement; and Cotlove, Ernest. *Clinical Laboratory Computerization.* Baltimore, Ohio: University Park Press, 1971.

Medical Computer Industry. Creative Strategies Incorporated: Palo Alto, Calif. 1971.

Souder, James J.; Clark, Welden E.; Elkind, Jerome I.; and Brown, Madison B. *Planning for Hospitals.* Chicago: American Hospital Association, 1964.

9

An Approach to Hospital Systems

INTRODUCTION

We have attempted to avoid excessive editorial comment throughout this text. It has seemed out of place in a book designed primarily for teaching purposes. With few exceptions, we have described factual conditions in the hospital as our experience and research have indicated them to be. Those few exceptions, however, since they were critical of some serious efforts in building hospital data processing systems, have left us with an obligation to provide suggestions for improvement. Thus, in this last chapter we depart from our circumspect treatment and develop a relatively new approach to hospital information management.

Criticizing previous efforts can be an interesting exercise, but is somewhat sterile if the analysis does not lead to some alternative suggestions. This chapter will be devoted to such a suggestion. An approach to what could become a total information system for a hospital will be described. By "approach" is meant the minimum necessary to do the jobs now recognized as essential, while leaving both room for expansion and capacity for eliminating functions as they become obsolete without redesigning the basic system structure. Notice the stress on "could become." Notice too that the discussion concerns an approach to a system design, not a finished plan.

In the following paragraphs we will propose a system design plan based on computer and communications hardware, programming methods, and operating procedures that have been proved effective in other commercial and institutional areas. The plan will be sensitive to the complexities of hospital information-processing problems as we have described them here and will maintain a healthy humility and respect for the attempts made by others.

At the same time, we will admit to a widespread dissatisfaction on the part of hospitals generally toward the accomplishments of data processing in their field. The successes of the computer in other industries have fostered a perhaps naïve expectation of similar successes when applied to the problems of health care information processing. As we have seen, the hopes have been realized only in a few narrow areas, and then only at great expense. The reasons for failure are many, and the excuses are still more numerous. They may be boiled down to two basic and related problems.

First, neither the hospital nor data-processing professionals have understood the problems to be treated on the one hand and the capabilities of the computer on the other. They have seldom spoken the same language.

Secondly, there has been a tendency on the part of vendors to sell and administrators to buy a "turn-key" system that will solve their particular problem in the most general way. This relieves the vendor from the efforts of truly learning the intricacies of the problem; and it relieves the hospital of getting deeply involved, of hiring competent people, or even of understanding the changes the computer will bring.

We make no pretense to solving these problems in one giant step. In the next few pages we will outline an approach that shows promise. The technical and economic realities of computers must still be assimilated before any approach will be successful.

BASIC PRELIMINARIES

One point should be crystal clear from all our previous discussions. The information-processing task for a hospital is impossible to define in any comprehensive closed sense because of its instability. We have seen that the data needed today may be useless tomorrow as medical research modifies medical practice. In our opinion, one of the reasons why "total" systems have achieved less than total success has been a failure to build in the flexibility required to grow with this inherent instability.

Another reason has been the readiness to depend upon a single large general purpose computer to handle communications, real-time, and batch jobs in a multiprogramming environment. There may be a computer built someday with the capability of performing these tasks economically, but that day has not arrived. The cost of systems using this approach runs from $40,000 to $80,000 per month for a 300-bed hospital, an amount few hospitals can afford.

Every functional part of a computer system, as well as the overall system itself, must be cost effective upon installation and must remain cost effective as long as it remains active. It is, however, most important to recognize that the business of a hospital is to save lives and prevent suffering. Therefore, "cost" has many facets beyond the usual monetary considerations. In an economic sense, the whole practice of medicine is of doubtful cost effectiveness; it might well be cheaper to let sick people die rather than keep them alive at tremendous investment of time and equipment. But medicine measures cost in terms of lives saved and pain alleviated.

Not everything that can be computerized should be computerized. Only if automation brings with it significant advantages, either economically, operationally, or medically, should it be the method of choice. Many functions do not need the speed and accuracy of computer processing. Many other areas do not have sufficient data volumes to justify the expense. Moreover, some functions lose valuable psychological benefits if they are dehumanized by computerization.

The problem of integrating new computer advancements into an already functioning system is not unique. Large scale telephone systems face this problem, since any new hardware such as electronic switching gear or two-way television equipment must be compatible, at least in a message transmission sense, with the oldest electromechanical relays still operative in the system. It is neither convenient nor economical to change everything at once every time an advance in technology occurs.

There is no magic in the solution of this problem. It consists of total commitment to three fundamental design characteristics, modularity, specialization, and compatibility. Every subsystem in the system design is built to stand alone, interacting only at the I/O level. Even when two or more functions are performed by the same piece of hardware, care is taken to see that the functions maintain their independence. Thus modules may be added, discarded, or exchanged without disruption of other modules, again except on an I/O level. Specialization is a natural result and corollary to modular design: it is easier to design modules to do one specific job than to integrate dissimilar functions into one module. Finally, hardware and software compatibility, especially at the I/O interface points, is of utmost importance. It can be accomplished by setting and maintaining programming and electronic standards for all I/O equipment and software. We will insure in what follows that the system design is based upon compatible, specialized modules.

Before we proceed with a description of the new system approach, let us diverge for a few paragraphs to discuss two topics of importance to the design that may be new to the nonspecialist. These are data base management and the minicomputer.

DATA BASE MANAGEMENT

Much has been written lately of this new concept in the management of information. Various names have been used—data bank, integrated files, data base, and so forth. They all refer to an information-processing technique that reduces or eliminates entirely the collection, input, and storage of redundant and repetitious data. This significantly reduces data input and storage costs and, in addition, preserves inherent data relationships.

Data base management techniques are predicated on three assumptions: (1) that as far as possible data should be collected and stored only once; (2) that all data concerning a business or institution should be recorded in central, integrated, and interrelated files; and (3) that the relationships between classes of stored data are seldom predictable in advance and thus that the storage and retrieval system must be capable of modifying relationships dynamically. This is an oversimplified view, but it will suffice for our purposes here.

Let us examine what the above assumptions imply in a hospital environment. First, we require that the name, address, services performed, charges, results, and so forth, relating to a given patient should be input once and recorded in one location for use by all departments in the hospital. As an example, consider the typical request for a laboratory test. We may recall from chapter 6 the sequence of events: The doctor writes an order; the nurse or clerk records the order in her ward log and fills out a lab ticket; the lab clerk logs in the test, patient identification, and lab work station; the lab technician performs the test and records the results in four places—the lab records, the patient's medical record, a business office copy, and a copy for the physician. Then the business office records the charges in yet another set of files. This single lab test may generate eight or more separate entries to unrelated files kept independently, yet containing the same basic information.

In a data base environment, the doctor's order would be entered by a clerk into the computer system. At that point the data base management program would record the identifying data, the source of the request, and the test desired; post the charges; and maintain a lab utilization file—all in an interrelated format allowing for references to the data either by test type, doctor i.d., patient i.d., lab work station, or any other key desired by the user.

There is more involved here than a simple reduction in the amount of writing and quantity of data being stored. To be truly meaningful, an item of information must be related to other items. Information has a structure, an internal coherence that should be reflected in the method of storage. Some methods tend to obscure these relationships. Anyone who has tried to relate a statement or detailed bill to the patient's medical record can attest to this fact. The data base concept was designed to preserve the inherent relationships between various pieces of information.

We shall leave to the user the exact form these concepts will take in the system. At this point, we can only say that the hospital data base consists of multiple files, on various kinds of storage media, containing all permanent and semipermanent data supplied by all hospital functions. The exact content of the files, what data is kept and how long, will depend on medical and management decisions and will vary considerably as the system is used.

MINICOMPUTER TECHNOLOGY

So-called minicomputers were developed to meet the need for low-cost, high-reliability, industrial process control automation. They were built to operate virtually unattended for long periods under conditions of extreme temperatures, moisture and dust, corrosive gases, and extreme vibrations—any of which would render their larger cousins inoperable. Their designers were more successful than they had hoped. With proper software, minicomputers can perform virtually all the tasks of their larger, more expensive counterparts, and at much lower costs. A recent article in *Electronics* (March 29, 1971) states that "for instance, eight 16-bit machines with 1-microsecond cycle times and costing $10,000 each might for some purposes give as good a performance, when suitably interconnected, as a machine in the $1 million class, with 64-bit words and a 500-nanosecond cycle time." Of course, there are tasks for which the larger machine is a better and more economical choice—such jobs as heavy engineering calculations, very large data base management, or extremely high data traffic. However, these are not the problems encountered in our hospital information system. The three vital factors for hospital and medical hardware usage are: (1) high reliability, (2) ease of backup in the event of failure, and (3) ability to perform the required tasks economically; that is, cost effectiveness. On all counts, the minicomputer has demonstrable superiority over the larger machines.

Reliability. Large computer mainframe manufacturers refuse to discuss reliability in any meaningful way, but a glance at the cost of the maintenance agreements is a good indication, as are the number of hours of preventive maintenance and the actual recorded downtime of large installations, the total of which may be 15 percent or more of the leased time. Minicomputer manufacturers are proud of their records; a quick look shows why. All major minicomputer manufacturers exceed military reliability specifications. In fact, some are achieving better than 7,000 hours mean time to failure, though they are somewhat more conservative in their quotations. This kind of reliability is not accidental. It is achieved by an exhaustive burn-in and testing procedure and by very thorough quality control and assurance methods. It is possible to apply these procedures to the manufacture of larger machines. However, with many more parts to test, the cost becomes prohibitive; and customers have not demanded it.

Backup. For extremely sensitive areas such as patient monitoring, diagnostics, and laboratory, there is yet another way of assuring reliability. If the same kind of hardware is used for business and accounting as well as medical applications, it is possible to interconnect these machines with electronic switches. Thus, if a failure on the medical computing side occurs, the business applications could be automatically interrupted, and the business computer would perform the medical task until maintenance could be completed, at which time the business applications would continue processing. The medical activity would lose at most a few seconds, and through proper program interrupt procedures the business program could proceed without any problems.

However, any piece of equipment as complex as a digital computer will eventually fail. When it does, it must be put back into working order quickly. This is especially important in a medical environment. Here, too, the minicomputer shows definite advantages. The miniaturization of the electronics and the low cost make it practical to keep a set of printed circuit boards having the complete circuitry of the system in stock. The maintenance procedure becomes the simple task of discovering which of four or five boards contains the problem area, and exchanging the board. Thus, the user can be back in operation in a matter of minutes. Contrast this with the hours, and sometimes days, required to locate the difficulty in a discrete-electronics conventional computer.

Cost Effectiveness. Three factors enter into the cost of computer hardware. These are purchase price or lease cost; reliability or maintenance cost, including such factors as ease of maintenance, percentage of downtime, and so forth; and cost of operation, particularly personnel. The purchase or lease of hardware to perform similar tasks can be a factor of ten less for minicomputers than for the larger machines. Factors of three to five are common. We have discussed the great advantages of minicomputer reliability and the ease with which minis are maintained. The operation of minicomputers does not require highly skilled operators. Simple, virtually unattended operation is one of the design features of the mini. Of course, hardware is only part of the cost of a computer system. One of the mini's few disadvantages is the relative lack of software. We shall return to this important point later.

SYSTEM ARCHITECTURE

With these convictions in mind, let us go on to consider a basic configuration of hardware and software, consistent with today's technology, yet leaving room for growth. The architecture to be proposed here is shown in functional block form in figure 9.1. There are three central modules and any number of outlying interacting modules. The three central modules are the data base, the data management system, and the data communications control system. Each of the modules on the periphery would be responsible for its special area of interest

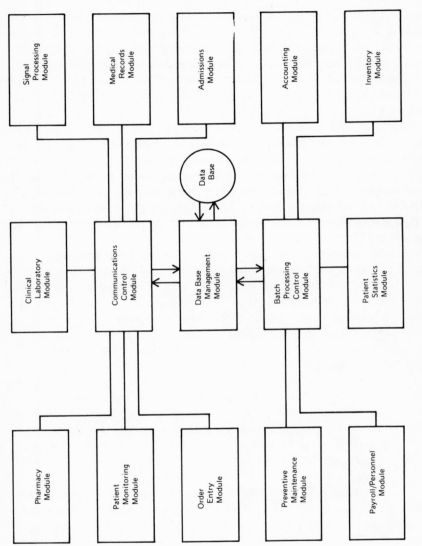

Figure 9.1   Hospital information system approach

157

and for assuring the proper input of data to the central files. Some volatile data could be stored at the module level for rapid access.

The data base, as we indicated in the previous pages, contains two kinds of data, volatile information and permanent information. These terms are, of course, relative. In practice there would be all gradations of permanence and volatility. The storage medium would be chosen on the basis of degree of permanence and on required response time. Accounting information is seldom required in real time; in fact, hours or days are sufficient response time for most of it. Patient monitoring data, on the other hand, may demand millisecond response. These factors obviously affect the implementation of the data base in major ways.

The data base management module is a hardware/software system that accepts data and/or store-retrieve commands in a standard format from the data communications control module. The hardware can be chosen from a group of minicomputers, numbering perhaps ten at present, whose memory speeds approximate one microsecond and whose instruction set supports list processing in a sophisticated and efficient manner. The software might be based upon one of the Disk Bill of Material Processor designs or might be written especially to take advantage of the properties of the chosen hardware.

The data communications control module must support data communications of two basic kinds, requests by one of the modules to store or retrieve certain data and the data to be operated upon. The communications module would interpret requests, store data in an active buffer, and feed both data and interpreted requests as instructions to the data management module. Another function of the data communications control module is the management of priority, resource allocation, and the loading of sequence control programs into the peripheral module processors when needed.

Since these modules are vital to the rest of the system, it might be advisable to provide continuous backup to the data base management and data communications control modules in the form of parallel processors. Alternatively, the most vital peripheral processors could be provided with emergency stand-alone capabilities, to be used only when the central modules are down. A careful trade-off study of cost and performance should be conducted before this decision is made.

The peripheral modules consist of computers with input/output hardware appropriate to their specific tasks, along with a special communications connection to the central modules. These peripheral modules operate independently of the central modules in most cases. The exceptions are program sequence control operations and emergency equipment failures in the central modules. It might be possible to install such modules as pharmacy, clinical laboratory, or accounting functions, each on its own computer or sharing where appropriate, before the central data base and management modules are complete; but any peripheral functions must be designed with eventual integration in mind. Therefore, the central modules should be designed, at least with respect to I/O requirements, so that compatibility with the other modules is assured.

Economic realities being what they are, it is likely that most hospitals will tend toward patient billing, cash control, and payroll as the first areas for automation, with clinical lab functions running a not-too-close second. Let us postulate a phased implementation plan using these ground rules.

IMPLEMENTATION

The installation of a computer-based information system is a large undertaking. The complexities of forms and procedures design, data collection, training, programming, data conversion, site preparation, and so forth, can be staggering to a hospital accustomed to manual methods. The tasks are best accomplished by careful planning, a phased approach to implementation, thorough checking as each task is completed, a period of parallel pilot operation, and the deep involvement of hospital management and personnel at each step in the project. The usual tasks to be accomplished fall naturally into four phases: (1) study and planning, (2) analysis and design, (3) implementation and planning, and (4) testing and pilot operation. The reader will recall the comments made in the previous chapter as we describe these phases.

Study and Planning

The study and planning phase should precede any peripheral module design or installation. It is vital that overall goals and plans be coordinated with the activities of each individual area; otherwise, the result is chaos. Two tasks are involved in this phase.

Task 1. A study should be made of hospital data-processing goals and their relation to the overall goals of the institution. Facilities, both existing and planned, must be surveyed in order to project data-processing loads. A long-range plan should be developed for the automation of selected administrative and medical application areas, all planning tasks to be performed in conjunction with hospital management and medical staff.

Task 2. A detailed implementation plan must be developed for each project identified in the long-range plan, including priorities, schedules and completion dates, manpower requirements, funding levels, and specific objectives. These plans are based on the design of the central modules. All items here are tentative until a complete analysis of each application can be performed. This task is intended to aid in the systems design work and to help management choose between alternatives.

Analysis and Design

The analysis and design phase follows logically the efforts initiated in phase one. The tasks in this phase utilize the planning information from phase one as a guide in the analysis of the systems to be implemented, in the order of priorities specified. The result of the analysis is a set of system design specifications for all planned applications. These specifications detail the exact characteristics of the central modules and the requirements for implementation of each of the applications in question. This phase continues throughout the life of the project, developing specifications, turning them over to hospital management for review, and moving on to the next application indicated. Several areas may be assumed to be of high priority.

Task 3. Source Data Collection System Design. This task will develop a method of data capture for admissions and discharge data, laboratory, X ray, central supply and pharmacy charges, room charges, credits, insurance data, and so forth, that is cost effective and quality controlled.

Task 4. Forms Design. The systems analyst will concentrate on the preparation of preliminary forms design specifications and layouts for those special purpose forms that may be required for source data input and special output reports, such as patient statements and collection bills.

Task 5. Report Content and Formats. Hospital personnel will develop preliminary report descriptions and prepare preliminary formats, utilizing data collected in task 1. The formats and content must conform to standards where industry-accepted formats and specific forms are required, such as those for Medicare (that is, SSA 1453c). These will be reviewed and approved prior to incorporation into the system.

Task 6. Business Systems Design. Several business and accounting applications are of such general and universal need that we recommend their immediate implementation. These include patient accounting, general ledger, property management, preventive maintenance, and management reporting functions.

Task 7. Medical System Design. There are many medical applications possible in a hospital setting. One of the values of this approach is the use of identical hardware and basic support programs for all applications, both business and medical, while leaving dedicated equipment in those areas requiring extreme reliability or real time operation.

Implementation and Training

Implementation and training have been included together in phase three because they go together in terms of personnel, timing, and documentation. The people involved in implementing a system are clearly those best suited to instruct others in its use. Furthermore, some of the documentation generated in implementation is exactly what is needed, with a few pedagogic additions, for training hospital personnel. Finally, it is obvious that the implementation task will be fruitless if the hospital is not prepared through personnel training to use it on completion.

Task 8. Programming and Check-out. This effort represents the software integration of the programs into their respective system modules and their interface with the data base management system. The fully integrated system should undergo rigorous testing prior to installation of on-site hardware. The programs to be implemented are determined by management according to the priorities set in task 1.

Task 9. Procedure and System Operation Manuals. The systems analyst will develop draft procedures covering data collection, audit control, input preparation, error correction, and so forth. These procedures will then be coordinated with hospital management for final typing and publishing of the procedures in established formats. The systems analyst will also develop and supply a definitive operating manual with simple, easy-to-follow instructions on every aspect of the system. Operating instructions will be linked to the procedure manual to help reduce error potential; each program will have a run diagram and other illustrations to facilitate both training and continued operation.

Task 10. Training. Hospital management should select the various individuals currently working in the business office that will be candidates for learning to operate the computer and perform data control check tasks. These individuals will start hands-on training as soon as the hardware is installed. The analyst should conduct, where necessary, training and orientation sessions for hospital personnel, including the nursing, administrative, and medical staffs. In addition, he should conduct management orientation sessions to familiarize them with the new reports.

Task 11. Site Preparation. This task will commence at the same time as task 1 with the development of a site plan for the installation. (It should be noted that other than the space required for the disk drives and printers and two 19-inch panel racks, this space is not much different from that required for several billing machines.) The site plan should include location of clerical personnel required to prepare input data and operate the computer. Minicomputers are designed with fully integrated circuitry, so that no significant change in air-conditioning load or overall power requirements is anticipated.

Task 12. Hardware Installation and System Test. The hardware should be scheduled for installation sufficiently prior to the system phase-over date to permit thorough check-out of all components and interface equipment. Standard system test procedures developed by the manufacturer will be performed, and trouble-free performance will be achieved prior to the final testing phase of the system. Approximately 30 days of testing must be performed prior to total data conversion.

Task 13. System Integration. This task is devoted to the design, fabrication, and testing of any unique electronic circuitry required to connect the desired peripheral components, such as card readers, printers, disk drives, tape drives, and so forth, to the computer's central processing unit (CPU). Occasionaly, the interface equipment available from the manufacturer is suitable, but more often considerable savings can be realized by building special purpose hardware. These interface systems should be checked out both prior to and during system test.

Task 14. Data Conversion. The good systems analyst should be experienced in the problems of accounts receivable conversion and the audit control procedures required to assure smooth phasing from a manual system to a computerized system. He will work closely with the accounting staff in planning the conversion. Audit checks must include definitive batch control over each part of the conversion process.

Testing and Pilot Operation

The final phase is the testing and pilot operation of the system prior to full operation. During this phase, a complete management review will be conducted on all parts of the completed system. Hospital personnel and staff members will examine each procedure, form, report, and application to assure that the system is performing its intended functions. Following this review, an extensive system test will be performed to determine that the total system operates properly. Upon completion of system tests, a pilot operations period will commence, with the new system running in parallel with the current one for a period of 30 to 60 days. This provides an opportunity for all operating departments to become familiar with the new system and procedures and shake out any errors. The phase-over process is accomplished with full audit control over all data-handling functions.

Task 15. Management review consists of a detailed examination of the entire system flow from source data collection to output reports to determine that all forms, procedures, reports, and computer applications are in accordance with previously established criteria. The review process will be conducted by hospital personnel to assure that the system is performing its intended functions.

Task 16. System test is a vital part of the implementation process. Specific tests are conducted to determine that the system processes normal data correctly, using discretely designed test data. Upon verification of accuracy, erroneous and test data with deliberate errors are entered to assure correct system detection of all parameters. Subsequently, various catastrophic system failures are simulated to determine proper system restart capability.

Task 17. Pilot Operation. This task begins with the conversion of existing data to the new system under strict conversion procedures with tight audit control to assure an accurate transition and parallel operation with the existing system for a period of 30 to 60 days. For those applications where no previous system or data exist for conversion, strict audit and data verification procedures are established to monitor the operation in order to assure accuracy. These special procedures are in effect for up to 60 days. The pilot operation period is also used to verify the training process and to eliminate areas of confusion that may arise with the hospital staff and is part of the continuing training effort commenced in task 10.

The above plan assumes that the hospital would prefer and can afford to attempt a completely integrated (though not total) system in one step. Many hospitals are not in a position to do this. For these institutions, an alternate schedule must be provided. What follows is a suggestion for such a schedule.

Stage 1. Design data base and data management system input and output characteristics. The file layouts and content and the maintenance and retrieval methods can wait, but I/O characteristics are essential.

Stage 2. Install a small general purpose computer to perform business and accounting tasks. Design all software to be compatible at the I/O level with the data base design. With the forms and procedures interface, this business system may require six months or more to install.

Stage 3. Subsequently, or concurrently if the staff and funds are available, install a special-purpose mini for clinical laboratory data collection and reporting. How much analog-to-digital and process control activity is implemented depends on the individual case, but at a minimum the system should do result report printing and provide charge data input for the business system. The I/O for these and any other functions should be compatible with the data base design.

Stage 4. Stage 3 may be repeated for any number of medical applications. Stage 2 may also be repeated to include purchasing and inventory control, general ledger, accounts payable, and so forth.

Stage 5. At some point, it will become necessary and desirable to implement the data base system. This is a big step that must itself be composed of separate stages; file design, storage and retrieval programming, access language design, and so forth. It must be decided if direct communications will be implemented; and if so, these programs must be written. It is suggested that each area or function be implemented one at a time and that a start be made perhaps with the business functions. Some functions may remain outside the central system for some time. Others will require almost immediate integration.

Three things should be said about what the above suggested system is not. First, it is not a panacea for all the ills of the hospital or even all its information-processing ills. Nor is the system a solution for everyone. A hospital contemplating the installation of a computer system must consider cautiously the resources available and the alternatives open to it. One important point to consider is the effect the computer may have on well-functioning personnel.

Some hospitals have installed expensive, sophisticated systems, only to find that lack of acceptance by hospital staff had doomed the project before it got started. The hospital may find also that the expenses do not stop with the computer and the personnel directly associated with its operation. Often, the changes required to keep the computer functioning properly must be accompanied by other equipment and procedural changes, which affect other areas, and so on, until the cost of the simple computer project has multiplied several times. For the right hospital with the right staff, the right kind of computer system can be of great value. The system described above is one of many possibilities, a better one than others, I submit, for some hospitals.

Secondly, it is not a revolutionary approach to data processing. All the pieces have been utilized successfully in one or another hospital system, and the whole approach has been tried in other industries. It is a straightforward extension of proved techniques, and its only claim to originality lies in the area of application. I predict that several commercial vendors and systems houses will be utilizing these concepts before the end of the decade, even if they never read this book. Given the constraints of funding and the data-processing requirements, it is an immanently logical approach.

Finally, the system is not one that will install itself, as many of the available systems will. The hardware installation provides few serious difficulties outside of some interface design, but the software is another problem. I know of no vendor of minicomputers that provides any significant portion of the programs required for the job. Few, if any, hospital business packages are available on minis, and no data base management software of the type required can be found. Two choices present themselves for the hospital desirous of immediate installation, vendor assistance, or a consulting firm. There are pros and cons for both choices, and the hospital will have to evaluate the alternatives for themselves. The other option, hiring a staff with competence in the required areas, is really unavailable to all but the richest hospital or one connected with a university. This kind of professional does not come cheap, and his usefulness for tasks beyond basic system design is questionable.

These disclaimers are not intended to scare a hospital away from data processing; but too often in the past computer-marketing people have painted a rosy picture of inexpensive, error-free performance awaiting the lucky hospital that installs an XYZ computer system. There are benefits, and there are grave dangers. It is only honesty not to understate either.

THE FUTURE

Where do we go from here? What can we as computer professionals expect and what can the hospital expect concerning data-processing requirements and solutions? One possibility is for the many systems currently available to continue to grow along their indicated path. Thus, the approach I suggested could continue to grow along the lines of its current design. This would mean expansion of the central data storage, perhaps a faster access system, and more sophisticated communications equipment as the present gear becomes overloaded. The peripheral areas could be handled for the foreseeable future on presently available minis. This method of growth would be satisfactory for many hospitals, at least at the present state of technology.

Another possibility is that of replacing the multiple processor architecture with a single large machine at some point in time. Unless the costs and the reliability of large systems improve significantly, I do not see this as a realistic possibility in the next few years.

Finally, another development might be the appearance of regional medical data bank installations. The effect of this could be to reduce the size of the in-hospital data base, while increasing the communications load. A similar effect would occur if the reporting requirements of the various third-party agencies change significantly.

All these future possibilities make the flexibility of the suggested system design a valuable asset; that is, the design meets the functional requirements and criteria likely to be imposed by clinical and administrative personnel as they attempt to satisfy the information needs of the modern medical center. We have seen that the hospital is an involved complex of over 35 departments, including administration, nursing, intensive care and treatment areas, laboratory facilities, and so forth. The information flow pattern that integrates this complex entity has been the subject for countless books and articles, including this one. All these treatments of the subject, again including the present one, have failed to provide definitive standards by which the design of a hospital information system may be certified to meet the requirements of some major set of hospitals.

The current approach has been conceived for the purpose of padding the bet; no matter what standards are chosen, the system approach should be valid, given economic viability.

Index